Acing the Hepatology Questions on the
GI Board Exam
THE ULTIMATE CRUNCH-TIME RESOURCE

BRENNAN M. R. SPIEGEL, MD, MSHS, FACG

Chief of Education and Training, UCLA
Division of Digestive Diseases

Program Director, UCLA
Gastroenterology Fellowship Training Program

Director, UCLA
Center for Outcomes Research and Education (CORE)

Associate Professor of Medicine,
David Geffen School of Medicine at UCLA
Los Angeles, California

HETAL A. KARSAN, MD, FACG, FACP
Clinical Assistant Professor of Medicine,
Emory University

Atlanta Gastroenterology Associates
Atlanta, Georgia

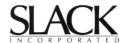

SLACK
INCORPORATED

www.slackbooks.com

ISBN: 978-1-55642-953-8

Copyright © 2012 by SLACK Incorporated

The procedures and practices described in this publication should be implemented in a manner consistent with the professional standards set for the circumstances that apply in each specific situation. Every effort has been made to confirm the accuracy of the information presented and to correctly relate generally accepted practices. The authors, editors, and publisher cannot accept responsibility for errors or exclusions or for the outcome of the material presented herein. There is no expressed or implied warranty of this book or information imparted by it. Care has been taken to ensure that drug selection and dosages are in accordance with currently accepted/recommended practice. Off-label uses of drugs may be discussed. Due to continuing research, changes in government policy and regulations, and various effects of drug reactions and interactions, it is recommended that the reader carefully review all materials and literature provided for each drug, especially those that are new or not frequently used. Some drugs or devices in this publication have clearance for use in a restricted research setting by the Food and Drug and Administration or FDA. Each professional should determine the FDA status of any drug or device prior to use in their practice. Any review or mention of specific companies or products is not intended as an endorsement by the author or publisher.

SLACK Incorporated uses a review process to evaluate submitted material. Prior to publication, educators or clinicians provide important feedback on the content that we publish. We welcome feedback on this work.

Published by: SLACK Incorporated
                   6900 Grove Road
                   Thorofare, NJ 08086 USA
                   Telephone: 856-848-1000
                   Fax: 856-848-6091
                   www.slackbooks.com

Contact SLACK Incorporated for more information about other books in this field or about the availability of our books from distributors outside the United States.

Library of Congress Cataloging-in-Publication Data

Spiegel, Brennan M.R., 1972-
  Acing the hepatology questions on the GI board exam : the ultimate crunch-time resource / Brennan Spiegel and Hetal A. Karsan.
     p. ; cm.
  Includes index.
   ISBN 978-1-55642-953-8 (pbk.)
  1. Liver--Diseases--Examinations, questions, etc. 2. Hepatology--Examinations, questions, etc. I. Karsan, Hetal A., 1971- II. Title.
  [DNLM: 1. Liver Diseases--Examination Questions. WI 18.2]
  RC845.S65 2011
  616.3'620076--dc23
                        2011025868

For permission to reprint material in another publication, contact SLACK Incorporated. Authorization to photocopy items for internal, personal, or academic use is granted by SLACK Incorporated provided that the appropriate fee is paid directly to Copyright Clearance Center. Prior to photocopying items, please contact the Copyright Clearance Center at 222 Rosewood Drive, Danvers, MA 01923 USA; phone: 978-750-8400; website: www.copyright.com; email: info@copyright.com

Printed in the United States of America.

Last digit is print number: 10   9   8   7   6   5

Acing the Hepatology Questions on the
GI Board Exam
THE ULTIMATE CRUNCH-TIME RESOURCE

DEDICATION

To my parents, who always encouraged me to "do the best you can, because nobody can ask for anything more, and you won't be satisfied with anything less." I've always remembered that.

—*Brennan M. R. Spiegel, MD, MSHS, FACG*

To my wife, Lina, who remains the most selfless person on this planet, and my children, Sonia and Rajan, who inspire me daily with their boundless enthusiasm. Iamque opus exegi. Om Shanti Shanti Shanti.

—*Hetal A. Karsan, MD, FACG, FACP*

CONTENTS

ACKNOWLEDGMENTS

The authors wish to thank the following individuals who provided images for this book:

- Stanley Dea, MD (Olive View–UCLA Medical Center)
- Francisco Durazo, MD (UCLA Medical Center)
- Alton B. Farris, MD (Emory University)
- Steven Hanish, MD (Emory University)
- Barbara Kadell, MD (UCLA Medical Center)
- Bobby Kalb, MD (Emory University)
- Dennis Jensen, MD (UCLA Medical Center)
- Charles Lassman, MD (UCLA Medical Center)

ABOUT THE AUTHORS

Brennan M. R. Spiegel, MD, MSHS, FACG is an Associate Professor of Medicine in the Division of Digestive Diseases, UCLA School of Medicine, and in the Division of Gastroenterology, VA Greater Los Angeles Health Care System. He is the section chief for Health Services Research at the UCLA Division of Digestive Diseases, and Chief of Education and Training in the UCLA GI Fellowship Training Program, which is amongst the largest GI Training Programs in the country.

Dr. Spiegel attended Tufts University where he majored in Philosophy and Community Health, and obtained his medical degree from New York Medical College. He received training in internal medicine at Cedars-Sinai Medical Center in Los Angeles, completed a fellowship in Gastroenterology at UCLA, and completed advanced studies in Health Services Research in the UCLA School of Public Health, where he received a master's degree in Health Services. He is board certified in Internal Medicine and Gastroenterology. He currently teaches in the Schools of Medicine and Public Health at UCLA.

Dr. Spiegel's research interests have focused on acid-peptic disorders, chronic liver disease, gastrointestinal hemorrhage, and functional bowel disorders such as irritable bowel syndrome and dyspepsia. He has performed research across a range of health services methodologies, including health-related quality of life measurement, survey design and administration, systematic review, meta-analysis, multivariable regression analysis, survival analysis, expert panel research, quality improvement, cost-effectiveness analysis, budget impact modeling, and use of clinical informatics to support decision making. He is a peer reviewer for numerous medical journals, and is on the editorial boards for the *American Journal of Gastroenterology* and *Clinical Gastroenterology and Hepatology*. He has contributed to the publication of more than 90 peer-reviewed papers, as well as numerous abstracts, book chapters, and monographs.

Hetal A. Karsan, MD, FACG, FACP is a Clinical Assistant Professor of Medicine in the Division of Digestive Diseases at Emory University School of Medicine in Atlanta. He is a gastroenterologist and hepatologist at Atlanta Gastroenterology Associates, one of the largest gastroenterology groups in the country, at which he is a partner. He is also a practicing clinician at Emory University.

Dr. Karsan attended Indiana University in Bloomington, Indiana, where he received his Bachelor of Science in Biology. While an undergraduate, he taught a course on Evolution and Diversity to fellow college students and won awards for undergraduate biomedical research from the Howard Hughes Medical Institute. He obtained his medical degree from Indiana University School of Medicine and went on to train in Internal Medicine at Boston University, where he completed his medical internship and residency. Dr. Karsan served as acting Chief Medical Resident while at Boston University. He completed fellowship at UCLA Medical Center, where he trained in gastroenterology, advanced interventional endoscopy, and transplant hepatology. While at UCLA, he won several awards and was nominated for the Teaching Fellow of the Year by the Department of Internal Medicine. He also sought formal training in clinical outcomes research at UCLA.

Dr. Karsan is active in numerous professional organizations and was elected as Fellow by both the American College of Gastroenterology and the American College of Physicians. In addition to contributions to various peer-reviewed manuscripts, abstracts, and book chapters, he also serves as a peer reviewer for medical journals and is on an editorial board. Dr. Karsan is board certified in internal medicine, gastroenterology, and transplant hepatology. He enjoys endoscopy and actively participates in clinical outcomes research. In his spare time, he enjoys playing sports, traveling, and spending time with his family.

PREFACE

You're holding the second book in the now-growing *Acing the GI Board Exam* series of review manuals. The first book, entitled *Acing the GI Board Exam: The Ultimate Crunch-Time Resource,* proved to be a well-received and unique approach to studying for the GI Board examination. Buoyed by positive reviews and seemingly satisfied readers of the first book, we opted to expand the series to the field of hepatology, a topic that constitutes 25% of the American Board of Internal Medicine (ABIM) GI Board examination. The purpose of this book is to complement the original effort by drilling deeper into liver knowledge for the GI exam, but not drilling so far that the result is diminishing returns. We have packed this volume with time-tested pearls that will help not only for the Board exam, but also for everyday clinical practice.

The first *Acing* book included a wide variety of liver questions. Here we provide new questions to round out the liver content likely to show up on a Board exam. We have minimized content overlap between the books to ensure this volume is unique from its predecessor. Between the two books, we now cover almost every major topic in liver disease, with a focus on the "tough stuff" liver vignettes you may not know the answer to (yet).

We've made every effort to write a modern, up-to-date liver textbook. The field of hepatology is constantly evolving; even hepatologists find it difficult to keep up with management guidelines for viral hepatitis, for example. We have tried to predict what might be on a Board exam 2 to 3 years from now, but have mainly kept to the traditional liver content that shows up in Board review. That said, we've not shied away from newer information. For example, if you're not yet aware of IL-28B polymorphism genotyping and its impact on hepatitis C management, then you should go read about it. We have included the use of the IL-28B polymorphism genotype test in this book, even though it's a relatively new discovery. In essence, we've attempted to reach a balance between novel information and time-tested knowledge, with an emphasis on the latter. We think we've hit the right balance, but you will be the ultimate judge.

Although the first *Acing* book was a single-author effort, the current book is a collaborative effort. Joining the project is Hetal Karsan, who brings experience not only as an academic hepatologist originally trained at UCLA and now practicing at Emory University, but also as a community-based general gastroenterologist and hepatologist with years of practical experience in a large GI practice group—Atlanta Gastroenterology Associates. Together, we've striven to ensure that this book maintains an appropriate balance between the academic theory and everyday clinical reality you need to know for success on the Board exam and clinical practice.

In the remainder of this Preface, we explain how the *Acing* approach works, and how we will try to get you where you need to be without going too far. We've maintained much of the same wording that was in the preface to the original *Acing* book, since the content is just as relevant to hepatology as it is to general gastroenterology. Then, in Chapter 1, entitled "Liver Disease on the GI Board Exam," we discuss issues specific to hepatology and describe how the current book aims to focus on liver knowledge of relevance to the general gastroenterologist.

At this point in your career you know a lot. It's been a hard-earned battle, but after years of reading books, sitting through lectures, and working with patients, you now have a pretty good sense of what is important and what is, well, less important. You are also busy, and your time is limited. So now that you have to study for Boards or prepare for a clerkship, your goal is to learn the information you don't know, not review the content you already do know.

Yet, for some reason, we all continue to practice an inefficient approach to studying for Board exams. This usually consists of comprehensively reviewing the entirety of a topic area without thinking about (a) whether we are adding incremental information to our pre-existing storehouse of knowledge, and (b) whether we are learning things that are actually on the examination. Presumably you have already done the painstaking work of learning the basics of your trade. Now you have to get down to business and ace a test. Those are two very different activities.

Yet the inefficient approach to Board review is perennially fostered by traditional "Board review" textbooks in which content areas are laid out in chapter-by-chapter (and verse) detail, fully laden with facts both high and low yield—both relevant and irrelevant to actual examinations. There's a time and place for the chapter and verse approach to learning your trade, but Board review crunch time probably is not it.

Board review books often present information that is not on the Boards (nor ever will be on the Boards) with information that is merely of personal interest to the chapter authors. That is, many Board review books suffer from the affliction of academia running roughshod over practical information. Such information is usually prefaced by the standard forerunners, like "Recent data indicate that...", or "Our group recently discovered that...", or "Although there is still a lack of consensus that...", and so forth. This kind of information is interesting and important for so many reasons, but is not relevant for Board review. When you are in crunch time, you should not have to read about pet theories, areas of utter controversy (and thus ineligible for Board exams), or brand new or incompletely tested data that are too immature for Board exams. You need to know about time-tested pearls that appear year after year—not cutting-edge hypotheses, novel speculations, new epidemiological oddities, or anything else not yet ready for prime time. Board exams are all about prime time.

The *Acing* books are different. They aim for the sweet spot between what you already know and what you do not already know (or have forgotten)—but that may be on the Boards. They try to avoid the lower extreme of information you have known since birth and the upper extreme of academic ruminations that are great for journal club or staying on the cutting edge, but that sit on the cutting room floor in Board exam editorial offices. You may find that you do know some of the content in this book, and if so, that's great. That means you're almost ready for the exam. But you will also find that you do not know (or have forgotten) much of what is in this book. And that's the point—you should be reading what you do not know, not reviewing content you already know well.

The information in this book has been culled from years of clinical practice and teaching Board review to our gastroenterology fellows at UCLA. We have come to realize that our fellows, who are among the "best of the best," know a lot about their specialty but are not necessarily ready for Boards. That's because we purposefully do not teach for Boards during everyday training—we instead teach the skills and knowledge that support rational and evidence-based decision making in clinical practice. Unfortunately, Board exams do not always tap directly into those skill sets. Great clinicians can do poorly on Board exams. And great test-takers can be suboptimal clinicians. We all recognize that it's primarily important to be a great clinician and secondarily important to be a great test-taker.

But with that caveat, it's still important to ace the Boards. Acing the Boards means that you ace not only the stuff you know, but also the "tough stuff" you may not yet know. This tough stuff tends to recur year after year.

This book consists of a series of "high-yield" vignettes on topics that are perennial Board review favorites—generally on the more difficult side—and full of pearls that may come in handy at Board time. All of these are originals; none are from an actual Board exam, naturally. But all have been endorsed, through an ongoing process of content development with our UCLA fellows and faculty, as being generally reflective of the content that might appear on GI Board exams. It goes without saying that we have no idea what will be on your particular Board exam—and even if we did, we sure as heck won't give you the answers in a book! Instead, we can make the more general statement that the content covered in this book is probably in the ballpark of things you should know to help you on the exam.

Here are some highlights of this book:

- **Focus on clinical vignettes.** We see actual patients in clinical practice. And, to the Board's credit, most Board questions are clinical vignettes. This book presents questions in the form of clinical vignettes, not sterile, fact-laden blocks of text.

- **Relatively short.** Most Board review books are better suited for arm curls than for rapidly and effectively teaching their content. Said another way, they are not "bathroom reading." Instead, most Board review books are read at a desk with a highlighter in hand. Unlike traditional didactic volumes, this book is big-time bathroom reading. You know, you sit down, open it up, and take in high-yield "tough stuff" in a hopefully entertaining format in short order. This is not a definitive text for comprehensive Board review, but a one-stop shop for high-impact content presented in a novel and interactive way. This book can be used in concert with longer volumes if you are looking for more extensive topic coverage.

- **Focus on stuff you don't know.** The goal of this book is for you to learn something new on every page, not to rehash what you already know. This book is relatively short, but it's dense with material you may not know yet. And that's the point—to learn stuff you don't know yet, not keep reading and re-reading stuff you've known forever.

- **Emphasis on pearl after pearl after pearl.** Students, residents, fellows, and even attendings love clinical pearls. And so do the Boards. After every vignette in this book, there is a pearl explicitly stated at the bottom introduced by the phrase, "Here's the Point!"

- **Random order of vignettes.** The Boards present questions in random order, not in nice, neat chapters. This book is meant to emulate the Board experience by providing vignettes in random order. It's a way to introduce cognitive dissonance into your learning by constantly switching directions. After all, patients appear in random order, so why not Board review material? If there's a specific topic you want to review, then you can look in the index to find the relevant pages. But again, keep in mind that this is not meant to be a treatise on any single topic, but instead a rapid-fire review of high-yield content.

- **No multiple-choice questions.** Multiple-choice questions are boring. They often test process of elimination more than knowledge and aptitude. When we teach Board review, we present a vignette, and then ask, "So what next?" Or, "What treatment will you give?" It's more entertaining and it's more realistic. A patient who comes into the office doesn't have a multiple-choice grid floating over his or her head in a hologram. So we find open-ended questions to be more engaging and interesting, even if the Boards emphasize multiple choice. We have no doubt that if you can get these questions right without multiple choice, you will most definitely get them right with multiple choice.

- **Emphasis on "clinical thresholds."** Many Board questions require that the test-taker has memorized some numerical threshold value. Like: "If an echinococcal cyst exceeds XX cm, then the risk of rupture is clinically significant and surgery is warranted." Or, "If the PMN count in ascites exceeds XX in cirrhosis, then the patient has spontaneous bacterial peritonitis and must be treated." And so forth. Throughout this book, we call these values *clinical thresholds*. They are emphasized through the vignettes and are separately cataloged toward the end of the book (pp. 215). The catalog is a one-stop shop for all the little numerical facts that everyone forgets but everyone needs to know. We often refer to this list ourselves because it's so easy to forget some of these critical threshold values.

- **Comprehensive yet parsimonious explanations.** Some books provide multiple-choice questions and give only the letter answer. The ABIM GI questions are a case in point. Other books provide short explanations. Still others provide full explanations but with information that isn't relevant. In this book we've striven to provide comprehensive answers that are also succinct, emphasizing the key clinical pearls. In other words, we've attempted to give you enough information to understand how to answer the questions correctly without overwhelming you with additional details. Board review isn't about ruminating forever about personal areas of interest—it's about cutting to the chase and keeping information on target.

- **Avoidance of mind-numbing prose.** Too many review books are boring as heck. They take away our will to live. This book is purposefully written in a manner that acknowledges that studying for Boards can be painful. We've tried to include interesting vignettes, provide answers that draw from real-life clinical experience, and avoid unnecessary jargon and excessive academic descriptions. We also love to use witty humor to keep your attention!

- **Emphasis on images.** Clinical medicine is a visual art, and GI and hepatology, in particular, are visual subspecialties. The Boards acknowledge this by including lots of questions with images. Many of the vignettes in this book are accompanied by carefully selected images designed to "bring the content to life" and aid in understanding the key points of the case.

This book was greatly enhanced by the feedback and input from current and former GI fellows at UCLA. We remain especially grateful to Benjamin Weinberg, who helped develop the title of the original *Acing the GI Board Exam* book, of which this is the second in the series. We would also like to thank Barbara Kadell

(Department of Radiology) and Charlie Lassman (Department of Pathology) at UCLA for providing key images to complement the text of this book, along with Alton B. Farris (Department of Pathology) and Bobby Kalb (Department of Radiology) at Emory University for additional images. These images greatly enhance the visual appeal and pedagogy of the text, and for that we are greatly appreciative.

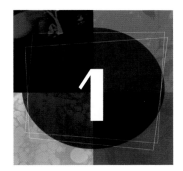

LIVER DISEASE ON THE GI BOARD EXAM

General Observations

As mentioned in the Preface, we have no idea what will show up on your Board exam. Nor do we have any knowledge about specific vignettes that have appeared on recent exams. We do, however, know which general content areas seem to be popular for Board review and which seem to be relatively de-emphasized. Of course, this may or may not correspond with what shows up on your exam. But with that caveat, here are some observations about general liver topics that tend to show up routinely.

Perennial Board Review "Favorites"

- **Pregnancy.** The Boards seem to love pregnancy. We pointed this out in the original *Acing* book and provided a range of vignettes in which pregnancy affects intestinal and hepatic function. But when it comes to preparing for the liver part of the exam, learning about pregnant women is absolutely necessary. So we have peppered this book throughout with the classics. These include acute fatty liver of pregnancy, HELLP syndrome, viral hepatitides in pregnancy, hyperemesis gravidarum, intrahepatic cholestasis of pregnancy, gallstones in pregnancy, route of delivery, and vertical transmission of viral hepatitis. When it comes to the Board exam, be sure to know this stuff.

- **Cirrhosis.** You just know cirrhosis will be all over the exam. But cirrhosis is a broad area, so it's helpful to focus on particularly high-yield topics within cirrhosis. In particular, be sure to know how cirrhosis affects the kidney. Common Board review topics include refractory ascites with an elevated creatinine, type I versus type II hepatorenal syndrome, mixed cryoglobulinemia with glomerulonephritis in hepatitis C liver disease, and medication-induced renal failure in cirrhosis. We have included several

Spiegel BMR, Karsan HA.
*Acing the Hepatology Questions on the GI Board
Exam: The Ultimate Crunch-Time Resource (pp 1-6)*
© 2012 SLACK Incorporated

vignettes about these topics (see the "cirrhosis/renal throwdown" in Vignettes 70-75). Other commonly tested areas in cirrhosis include hepatic encephalopathy, hepatopulmonary syndrome, specifics of ascites management, portal hypertension, management of esophageal varices, and evaluation and treatment of spontaneous bacterial peritonitis.

- **Drug-Induced Liver Injury (DILI).** With so many drugs, herbals, and other substances that can affect the liver, it's virtually a lock to see some DILI questions on the Board exam. Know what drugs cause microvesicular versus macrovesicular steatosis (covered in the first *Acing* book), and be able to recognize pathognomonic patterns of individual drugs. Classic Board review topics include the phospholipid-laden lysosomal lamellar bodies seen with amiodarone hepatotoxicity, antibiotic-induced cholestasis from trimethoprim-sulfamethoxazole, erythromycin, or amoxicillin-clavulanate, and autoimmune-type DILI from diclofenac, minocycline, nitrofurantoin, phenytoin, and propylthiouracil. Classic herbals that can affect the liver include kava kava, ephedra, mistletoe, and herbal teas. And don't forget about acetaminophen. Finally, remember that various illicit drugs can cause acute liver injury. We have addressed all of these plus many more in the "DILI Delight" section of the book (see Vignettes 14 to 22) and other vignettes.

- **Metabolic Liver Diseases.** It's almost a guarantee that you will be asked about Wilson disease, hereditary hemochromatosis (HHC), and α-1 antitrypsin (AT) deficiency. Just know these. Be sure to know classic "factlets" such as treat HHC before hepatitis C (HCV) in HCV-infected patients; low alkaline phosphatase (ALP) and hemolytic anemia are seen in Wilson disease; and PAS-positive globules accumulated in hepatocytes are seen in α-1 AT deficiency. We focus on these and many other facts you need to know in the metabolic liver disease vignettes in this book. For example, you will find the top 10 facts of Wilson disease in Vignette 36. We have also included characteristic micrographs of these classics. Images are important, and this book does not skimp on them.

- **Vascular Diseases Affecting the Liver.** Be sure to review Budd-Chiari syndrome, veno-occlusive disease (also called sinusoidal obstruction syndrome, or SOS), and nutmeg liver, seen in right heart failure. Also, with the variety of patients who present with hepatic bruits on physical exam, it's important to know the differential diagnosis for hepatic bruits, which includes acute alcoholic hepatitis, arteriovenous fistula, hepatic artery aneurysm, and so forth. We've got these covered.

- **Nutritional Deficiencies.** The American Board of Internal Medicine (ABIM) states that nutritional deficiencies compose a small part of the "general" category, which makes up 7% of the exam. Thus, you might expect only 1 or 2 questions about nutritional deficiencies. So it's not necessarily high-yield to learn all the nutritional deficiencies from the standpoint of total questions, but it is high-yield from the standpoint of the likelihood that these deficiencies will show up on the exam, even if in small numbers. Perennial Board review favorites include zinc deficiency, biotin deficiency, and selenium deficiency (cardiomyopathy). If you're in crunch time, it's almost a sure bet that spending 20 minutes on the deficiencies will yield at least a couple of correct answers. We have included a section called "Vitamin Power!" which reviews major vitamin deficiencies with a focus on fat-soluble vitamin deficiencies commonly seen in cholestatic liver diseases (see Vignettes 52-55).

- **Dermatological Manifestations of Liver Diseases.** This is a favorite Board review topic because it reminds all of us that we are internists first and subspecialists second. Moreover, it's easy to test this material because the content is set up for picture images. It's a high-yield activity to review all the major liver-dermatology links, including migratory necrolytic erythema in glucagonoma, porphyria cutanea tarda in HCV, and skin rashes from interferon and ribavirin therapy.

- **HCV Infection.** This is one example where the prevalence of the disease in the community appears to be matched by its prevalence on the examination. As with hepatitis B virus (HBV) treatment, HCV therapy remains a rapidly changing area, so you will generally be held accountable for older, well-supported facts, not recent innovations or cutting-edge data from the newest combination therapies (with some exceptions, noted in the book). Be sure that you can interpret responses to combination therapy with interferon and ribavirin, including knowing the definitions for rapid virologic response (RVR), early virologic response (EVR), sustained virologic response (SVR), slow responder, nonresponder, and null responder. We've got these definitions covered (see Vignette 64). We have also added a vignette covering prime-time information regarding the IL-28B genotype and how it predicts response to interferon and ribavirin therapy in genotype 1 HCV. We think this is important to know for the exam, even if it's relatively new.

- **HBV Infection.** Because you probably memorized the HBV serotype patterns back in medical school, we have not included a vignette on basic serologic patterns. But to succeed on the GI Board exam, you will need to know more nuanced details about HBV. Be acutely aware of how to manage HBV in pregnancy, what the differences are between various HBV genotypes, and how to manage acute HBV liver failure. Know the relationship between HBV and polyarteritis nodosa and between HBV and hepatocellular cancer. Learn about flares following anti-tumor necrosis factor (TNF) therapy or steroid administration. The treatment algorithms for HBV seem to vary all the time, and the existing guidelines are themselves inconsistent, so you should not be asked too much about treatment algorithms. But you should at least understand the impact of HBeAg status and how that might affect duration of treatment.

- **Nonviral Liver Infections.** When studying for the Board exam, it's easy to be lulled into the siren song of viral hepatitis. While you should study viral hepatitis carefully because it's very likely to show up on your exam, it's also important to focus on a number of other liver infections. Some classics include salmonella hepatitis (think temperature-pulse differential, rose spots, and a stepwise fever along with hepatitis), fascioliasis (a nasty disease, with an awesome case described in this book), echinococcal liver cysts (think sheepherder with "eggshell calcifications" on a liver cyst), schistosomiasis, clonorchiasis, and *Entamoeba histolytica* abscess (think "anchovy paste"). There are Board buzzwords for all of these conditions, and it will probably be worth it for you to link the buzzwords with the diagnoses. We will cover these topics throughout the book. But in the meantime, try to name the nonviral infectious diagnosis for each of the following buzzwords: Katayama fever, transverse myelitis, anaphylaxis after cystic rupture, undercooked fish, cyst filled with hydatid sand, tortuous tracks in liver on CT, contaminated freshwater plants, portal vein granulomas with fibrosis. If some of these have you stumped, stay tuned—all of these are covered in the vignettes, and we have pulled them together in a table of Board buzzwords with their associated conditions (see Table 44-1). That table is gold!

Generally De-Emphasized Topics

In contrast to the topics just discussed, other areas of hepatology have historically been de-emphasized in Board review. Of course, that does not mean that next year's exam won't be filled to the brim with these topics. And furthermore, "historically de-emphasized" does not mean absent from the exam altogether— just de-emphasized compared to other topics. Here are some topics that we think will probably get relatively short shrift on the exam (but who knows...?).

- **Liver Transplantation.** Hepatology is an exploding field, and the GI Board exam heavily emphasizes this field. In fact, the ABIM states that 1 in 4 Board questions pertains to hepatology. So, if you are not a big "liver fan," now is the time to become one because you have to know liver. But, there is a fine line between the hepatology that a general GI should know and the specialized knowledge that a full-fledged hepatologist should know. This is not a test for budding transplant hepatologists. There is a move afoot to better define the hepatology curriculum, and there is now a separate ABIM examination for transplant hepatology. Liver transplantation is a very specialized area that is generally reserved for "official" transplant hepatologists. It's not expected that community gastroenterologists know how to manage the intricacies of post-transplant patients. Pre-transplant issues, such as staging with the Model for End-Stage Liver Disease (MELD), are relevant to practicing GIs and are also on the Board examination. However, perioperative and postoperative transplant topics have not been heavily emphasized on the general GI examination. If you're in crunch time, it's probably low yield to start learning those topics, particularly if you have not already been exposed to post liver transplant patients in much detail. But know the basics: What is MELD? How is MELD used? What are the indications and contraindications to liver transplant? What are the criteria for hepatocellular carcinoma (HCC) and transplant eligibility? What is the most common de novo malignancy in the long term after liver transplantation (no, not lymphoma...)? and so forth. If you can answer these basic questions, then you should be well on your way to getting the basic transplant-related questions correct on the Boards. We covered these topics in the first *Acing* book and have added some additional vignettes in this book to round out these areas.

- **Nonbiliary Radiology.** You need to know basic cholangiograms, but the Board examiners should hopefully recognize that you are a gastroenterologist—not a radiologist. Even though GI and hepatology rely heavily on abdominal imaging in everyday clinical practice, it is expected that you will be working with radiologists when interpreting images. So, on the Board exam you should rarely, if ever, be given a radiograph without supporting information. There should be enough information in the vignette for you to piece together what is happening in the image, even if you cannot actually interpret the image. It's still useful to be able to recognize basic radiographic patterns (eg, ascites, subcapsular hepatic adenoma, spoked-wheel pattern of focal nodular hyperplasia [FNH], the difference between FNH and fibrolamellar hepatocellular carcinoma, and hemangiomas), but at this point you pretty much know what you know when it comes to liver imaging. It will be generally low yield to spend Board review crunch time carefully studying different CT, MR, or ultrasound images. If you are going to study images, we recommend spending time reviewing cholangiograms. For nonbiliary images, you should be able to rely on your general knowledge about imaging and couple that with your specific knowledge about liver diseases, since—as noted earlier—the accompanying vignettes should have sufficient data to allow correct answers even if you can't precisely interpret the provided image. With that said, we have included a wide variety of classic images in this book for several liver disorders (reprinted with permission from Barbara Kadell from UCLA, possibly the best GI radiologist to ever walk the Earth. Seriously, she is unmatched... once, she diagnosed breast cancer just by looking at the *cecum* of a KUB, and was dead right!). If you can interpret the images included in this book, then you should be well on your way to recognizing most of the major liver radiographs that might show up on a Board exam. We worked carefully with Dr. Kadell to select some of the highest-yield images we could think of. You will see them scattered throughout the text.

- **Pathology Interpretation.** Pathology interpretation is a fundamental skill for practicing gastroenterologists and hepatologists. Every biopsy we take needs pathologic interpretation, and the results almost always have important clinical implications. But at the same time, we are gastroenterologists and hepatologists, not pathologists. Similar to the radiology discussion, it's generally the case that Board questions tied to pathology results will provide sufficient information to answer the question without having to precisely interpret the histopathology. Undoubtedly, you need to know some basic patterns of histopathology: interface hepatitis with plasma cells in autoimmune hepatitis, "onion skinning" in primary sclerosing cholangitis (and other chronic cholestatic conditions), "florid duct lesions" in primary biliary cirrhosis, Mallory bodies, hepatocyte ballooning and portal inflammation in nonalcoholic fatty liver disease, among many others. But in each of these cases, the exam should provide concurrent clinical information, and you should be able to piece together the answer without being an expert in histopathologic interpretation. In situations where you are called upon to directly interpret a pathology slide, chances are the abnormality will be right under your nose and "classic"—not some strange variation. Leave it to the pathologists to be experts in interpreting fine degrees of separation between conditions. You should know the basics and be able to tie those basics to clinical information. We expect the Board will focus on the pathognomonic classics when it comes to requiring histopathologic interpretation. You will find many classic liver micrographs featured in this book (reprinted with permission from Dr. Charles Lassman from UCLA and Dr. Alton B. Farris from Emory University—both outstanding teachers and top liver histopathology experts)—we think we've got almost all of the classics covered.

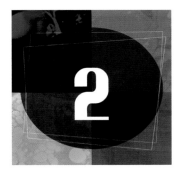

"Tough Stuff" Vignettes

In the pages that follow are 95 "tough stuff" vignettes. As described in the Preface, these have been culled from years of teaching Board review and practicing gastroenterology and hepatology and have been iteratively reviewed and vetted with our fellows at UCLA. As you go through these vignettes, keep the following points in mind:

- These are generally difficult. That is by design. You may nonetheless know the answers to many of the questions in these vignettes—a sign that you are well prepared for the exam. But if you cannot get them all right, that is fine, too. That's the whole point of this book—to ensure that you're gaining incremental information, not just reviewing content you already know. Keep in mind, however, that for every tough question that's in this book, there will be a bunch of "gimmies" on the exam. The entire Board exam won't be full of "tough stuff" questions. So don't get demoralized if you can't answer all of the questions in this book correctly. Rest assured that you already know most of the "gimmies" just by virtue of paying attention and learning during your clinical experiences.

- These are in completely random order—there is no explicit rhyme or reason. See the Preface for our rationale for this setup.

- The vignettes appear on one page, followed by one or more open-ended questions. The answers are provided on the next page. Before you turn the page, take a moment to really think about the answers. Even if you're not sure of an answer, at least take a moment to think about the potential differential diagnosis, or other information you might need to better answer the question. This form of active learning is more useful than merely flipping the page and reading the answer. Seriously... don't just flip the page until you've given the vignette at least a nanosecond of thought. The answer will be more meaningful if you've first struggled a bit to think through the vignette.

Spiegel BMR, Karsan HA.
*Acing the Hepatology Questions on the GI Board
Exam: The Ultimate Crunch-Time Resource (pp 7-214)*
© 2012 SLACK Incorporated

- After each answer there is a short section entitled "Why Might This Be Tested?" The purpose of this discussion is to emphasize why it's important to know the content of the vignette, *vis-à-vis* the Board exam in particular. It puts you in the mind of the Board examiners to better understand their potential reasoning, which might help you better remember the vignette.

- At the bottom of each answer page there is a box entitled "Here's the Point!" This summarizes the key issue or issues that appear on the page. If you are really in crunch time, at the very least make sure you know the "Here's the Point!" bottom line for each vignette. The "Crunch-Time Self-Test" on page 221 catalogs all of these factlets (and more) into a 135-question test that quizzes you on the key points from each vignette.

- Some of the answer pages also have a "Clinical Threshold Alert," followed by the presentation of an explicit clinical threshold (see the Preface for details). Sixty of these clinical thresholds are cataloged on page 215 for your convenience during crunch time.

Vignette 1: Severe "Transaminemia"

A 50-year-old man presents to the emergency room with a chief complaint of malaise. The following laboratory values are noted:

AST = 1200
ALT = 2100
LDH = 300

▶ **Without knowing anything else, what is the most likely diagnosis?**

▶ **Why?**

Vignette 1: Answer

This is acute viral hepatitis. You might wonder how 3 lab values and a single symptom would clinch this diagnosis. If so, it's worth taking some time to break down this short yet demonstrative vignette. It turns out that there's enough information here to narrow the diagnosis to acute viral hepatitis with a high degree of reliability. You certainly can't pinpoint the type of virus with this information alone, but you can at least posit an underlying acute viral infection.

First off, it's important to note that the serum aminotransferases, AST and ALT, are extremely high—both above 1000 U/L. This degree of "transaminemia" (not, by the way, "transaminitis," which literally means "inflammation of the transaminases" and makes no sense despite the term's deep penetration into common parlance) can occur only from a short list of conditions. When the AST and ALT are in the 1000+ range, think about the following potential causes: (1) acute viral hepatitis, (2) acute drug or toxin injury, and (3) shock liver. On occasion, an acute flare of autoimmune hepatitis or an acute bile duct obstruction (ie, common duct stone) can lead to aminotransferase levels over 1000, but that would be relatively uncommon. A wide range of other conditions can also cause hepatitis, but not with this degree of marked transaminemia.

A classic trick question is to describe an alcoholic who presents to the emergency department with an AST of, say, 2000 and an ALT of 1000, and then ask you to make the diagnosis. The usual first temptation is to diagnose acute alcoholic hepatitis and call it a day. Indeed, every med student knows that acute alcohol poisoning can present biochemically with an AST:ALT ratio of 2:1 (more on alcohol injury in Vignette 26), but not with enzymes in the 1000+ range. In fact, it's highly unusual for the AST to exceed 400 to 500 in the setting of pure alcoholic liver disease without some other hepatotoxin on board. So in an alcoholic patient who presents with a 2:1 ratio of AST to ALT but with liver enzymes in the 1000+ range, think about something else—like underlying acetaminophen toxicity in addition to acute alcoholic hepatitis.

Now, with a little more information, you could start to distinguish between underlying etiologies for severe transaminemia. For example, if the patient were in the intensive care unit and recently suffered a bout of pronounced hypotension, then shock liver would lead the differential diagnosis. If the patient had just eaten shellfish and turned yellow, then acute hepatitis A might be high on the list. If the patient had recently started a new herbal remedy recommended by a homeopathic healer, then toxin-mediated injury might be the diagnosis. If the patient had just consumed half a bottle of, say, Vicodin or Percocet, then acetaminophen injury would be highly suspected. If an obese, 40-year-old woman presented with acute biliary colic, then a common bile duct stone would be considered. And so forth. But you do not have any of that information here; this is a bare-boned question.

So, that should lead you to evaluate the LDH level. Recall that LDH has several forms and arises from not only the liver but also the heart, reticuloendothelial system, lungs, kidney, and striated muscles. So, it's all over the place and not very sensitive for liver disease, in particular. And it comes in 5 isoforms that, for the most part, are not routinely fractionated in everyday clinical practice. But the bottom line is that LDH is often included in metabolic panels and the information it provides is, on occasion, quite helpful. The LDH is elevated in this case, although it's not inordinately high. How can that help you narrow the diagnosis? The key is to evaluate the ratio of ALT to LDH. Serum LDH is especially high in the setting of hypoxemic liver injury ("shock liver") and in both toxin- and drug-induced liver injury. In these situations, both the aminotransferases and the LDH are high, with the LDH disproportionately high compared to the already high ALT. The ALT:LDH ratio is therefore low. In acute viral hepatitis, in contrast, LDH levels are not as high, so the ALT:LDH ratio tends to be much higher. In the original validation study of this concept by Cassidy and Reynolds (see the Bibliography in the back of this book), the mean ALT:LDH ratio for acute viral hepatitis was 4.65. In contrast, the ratios for hypoxemic liver injury and acetaminophen injury were 0.87 and 1.46, respectively. A cutoff of 1.5 distinguished acute viral hepatitis from hypoxemic, toxin-induced, and drug-induced hepatitis with a sensitivity of 94% and a specificity of 84%.

In the current vignette, the ALT:LDH ratio is 7.0. The high ratio argues strongly against hypoxemic, toxin-induced, and drug-induced liver injury, all of which tend to disproportionately elevate the LDH. That leaves acute viral hepatitis as the most likely explanation for the biochemical pattern. Fatigue is also supportive of viral hepatitis but is by no means specific. Although acute autoimmune hepatitis and bile duct obstruction can also drive the aminotransferases into the 1000+ range, acute viral hepatitis would be much more likely. When all of these factors are considered, it's reasonable to conclude that acute viral hepatitis is the best explanation for the marked transaminemia.

While we're on the topic of aminotransferases, it's worth reviewing a few other useful factlets about their use in diagnosing and managing liver disease. First, the degree of transaminemia is not predictive of the level of hepatic necrosis. That is, although aminotransferase levels in the 1000+ range can be intimidating, they do not necessarily portend a bad prognosis in and of themselves. This highlights the fact that ALT and AST are liver enzymes but are not liver function tests, or LFTs. For some reason ALT and AST are typically referred to as "LFTs" when, in fact, they do not measure liver function at all. They indirectly measure hepatocyte damage, but they do not provide insight into the functional deficit engendered by that damage.

This leads to the second point, which is to distinguish the aminotransferases from true LFTs, including albumin, INR, and total bilirubin. These lab values provide direct evidence of liver function and true prognostic information; they can predict, quite literally, whether a patient with advanced liver disease will live or die without a transplant. The aminotransferases simply cannot provide this information and are therefore not LFTs at all.

Third, it's notable that while the absolute aminotransferase levels do not provide prognostic information, their rate of decline may. In severe cases of acute liver injury, the ALT and AST values may rise quickly and subsequently fall even faster. This suggests a rapid burnout of the liver from overwhelming necrosis. When coupled with an abrupt rise in bilirubin and INR, a rapid drop in aminotransferase levels portends a bad prognosis. But that's enough factlets for now.

One final point in passing—the term *aminotransaminases* is now favored over the term *transaminases*, since it more accurately describes the function of the enzymes. But that will not be on a Board exam. And, quite frankly, we tend to switch back and forth when we use the terms.

Why Might This Be Tested? For the general gastroenterology exam, you will not be expected to know everything about hepatology, which is a burgeoning field. But you should certainly be able to interpret basic patterns in liver tests. Marked transaminemia is perfect for a Board question because the differential diagnosis is quite narrow, so the choices are limited. A Board question will likely give more information than what we have provided here, but knowing the relationship between ALT and LDH could help you answer a question more efficiently and reliably without getting too waylaid by the inevitable red herrings test writers like to pepper into vignettes. That was a mixed metaphor, but who cares? We're doctors, not English professors.

Clinical Threshold Alert: If the ALT:LDH ratio exceeds 1.5 in the setting of severe transaminemia, think acute viral hepatitis. If the ratio is lower, think about toxin-induced, drug-induced, or hypoxemia-induced liver injury.

Here's the Point!

When the aminotransferases enter the 1000+ range, think:
- **Acute viral hepatitis**
- **Shock liver**
- **Drug- or toxin-induced liver injury**

Here's the Point!

The ALT and AST are not LFTs. The "real" LFTs include:
- **Total bilirubin**
- **Albumin**
- **INR**

Vignette 2: Bloated With Bleeding Gums

A 46-year-old woman with morbid obesity had been successfully losing weight while on a monitored dietary regimen over the past year. However, she continued to experience abdominal bloating and increased abdominal girth despite the overall weight loss. Her primary care provider noted that all of her blood tests were normal on routine annual physical examination last month, but ordered an abdominal MRI to further evaluate the progressive abdominal bloating (Figure 2-1).

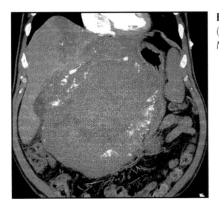

Figure 2-1. Abdominal MRI for the patient in Vignette 2. (Reprinted with permission of Barbara Kadell, MD, UCLA Medical Center.)

The patient subsequently presented to the emergency department with complaints of bleeding gums for the past week associated with a further increase in abdominal girth and pain, along with progressive jaundice. There was no history of trauma. Laboratory tests revealed the following: total bilirubin = 4.9, ALT = 51, AST = 62, INR = 2.2, hemoglobin = 7.2, platelets = 40,000, fibrinogen = 43 mg/dL (low), fibrin degradation products = 60 µg/mL (high), aPTT = 72 seconds (high). The patient received transfusions of various blood products and underwent emergent surgery, which resulted in resection of a large liver tumor (Figure 2-2).

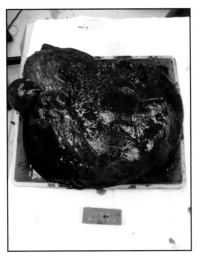

Figure 2-2. Large liver tumor resected from the patient in Vignette 2 (wow!). (Reprinted with permission of Steven Hanish, MD, Emory University.)

▶ *What is the diagnosis?*

Vignette 2: Answer

This is Kasabach-Merritt syndrome (KMS) associated with a giant (ie, humongous) cavernous hemangioma. KMS is a consumptive coagulopathy that can lead to disseminated intravascular coagulopathy (DIC). The syndrome was originally described in 1940 in a young child with a rapidly growing cutaneous hemangioma. KMS has also been recognized as a rare complication of giant hepatic hemangiomas. In this case, resection of the giant hemangioma cured the KMS-associated clotting and fibrinolysis.

Cavernous hemangioma is the most common benign tumor of the liver and has been found in nearly 10% of autopsies—so you may have one right now without knowing it. Hemangiomas are more common in women than men. They are usually noted incidentally and rarely require treatment. However, some of these can enlarge, and they are given the designation "giant" when they grow to more than 5 cm in diameter. These giant hemangiomas can lead to symptoms, including chronic pain from stretching Glisson's capsule, massive hepatomegaly, early satiety from gastric compression, jaundice from biliary compression, vascular compression, DIC, and even rupture! Indeed, a spontaneous rupture is a rare occurrence in giant hemangiomas, but it can have a disastrous outcome with a nearly 40% mortality rate. Treatment options for symptomatic giant hemangiomas include resection, transarterial embolization (enucleation), and even liver transplantation.

On gross examination, giant hemangiomas have a sponge-like, purplish appearance. Just look at that thing—it's an amazing lesion. Furthermore, hemangiomas may have regions of calcification, scarring, and intraluminal thrombosis. On microscopic examination, there are networks of blood-filled vascular spaces separated by thin, fibrous stroma (Figure 2-3).

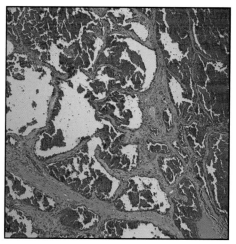

Figure 2-3. Micrograph of hepatic hemangioma demonstrating networks of blood-filled vascular spaces separated by fibrous stroma. (Reprinted with permission of Charles Lassman, MD, UCLA Medical Center.)

Because there is a significant risk of bleeding with biopsy of this type of lesion (obvious just by looking at the micrograph), the diagnosis of hemangioma is usually made on the basis of imaging alone without biopsy. On ultrasonography, these tumors appear as hyperechoic lesions with smooth margins. On contrast-enhanced CT or MRI, hemangiomas are well-circumscribed lesions with a characteristic progressive centripetal (from the periphery to the center) fill-in. If the diagnosis is still unclear after these imaging studies are conducted, then a technetium-labeled red blood cell nuclear scan can be employed as a noninvasive test to help clinch the diagnosis. With this scan, there should be increased uptake of the isotope within the lesion during the venous phase with retention on delayed images. Following diagnosis of a giant hemangioma, it's reasonable to perform follow-up imaging—especially if the lesion is subcapsular—since this location confers a higher risk of bleeding upon tumor enlargement. Otherwise, stable and asymptomatic lesions do not necessarily need to be followed.

Why Might This Be Tested? Since hemangiomas are the most common hepatic tumor, you should know their characteristics. Furthermore, you need to keep anatomic considerations in mind when determining a surveillance and treatment plan—good fodder for a Board exam. Incidental liver lesions are one of the most common reasons for consultation requests (either formal or curbside) that gastroenterologists will encounter, so you need to know about all the common liver tumors that arise. We cover most of these within this volume and the previous *Acing* book.

Here's the Point!

DIC + Giant hemangioma = Kasabach-Merritt syndrome

Vignette 3: Isolated Fundic Varices

A 62-year-old man with chronic alcoholic pancreatitis presents with 4 hours of large-volume hematemesis that began abruptly after drinking several beers. The patient does not have a history of cirrhosis. After stabilization in the emergency department, the patient undergoes urgent upper endoscopy, which reveals large varices in the fundus of the stomach (Figure 3-1). No esophageal or gastroesophageal junctional varices are noted.

Figure 3-1. Fundic varices. (Reprinted with permission of Dennis Jensen, MD, UCLA Medical Center.)

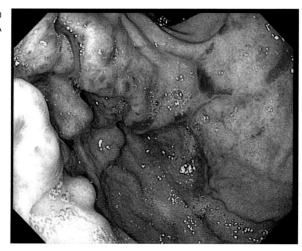

▶ **What might explain these endoscopic findings?**

▶ **How should this be treated?**

Vignette 3: Answer

These are isolated fundic varices resulting from an underlying splenic vein thrombosis from chronic pancreatitis. This vignette provides an excuse to review the anatomy of the portal circulation, which you need to understand in order to know why and how isolated fundic varices can form. Figure 3-2 provides a simplified depiction of the portal circulation—refer to this figure as you read the text that follows.

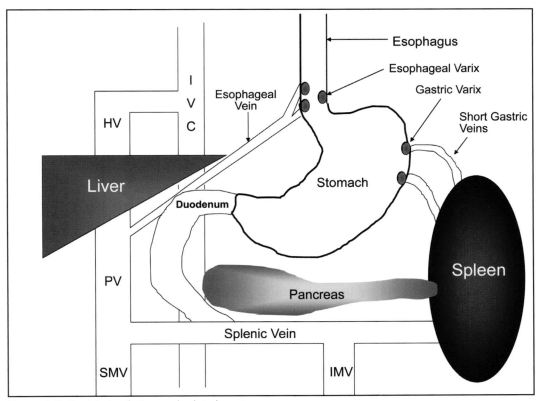

Figure 3-2. Portal circulation and related anatomy.

Recall that the portal circulation flows into and out of the liver via the portal vein and hepatic vein, respectively. The hepatic vein joins the inferior vena cava to return blood to the heart for recirculation. On the other side of the liver, the portal vein is formed by the confluence of the superior mesenteric vein and the splenic vein. The esophageal vein branches off the portal vein and heads toward a venous plexus surrounding the gastroesophageal junction. In the setting of cirrhosis, where there is intrinsic liver disease marked by portal hypertension, blood cannot push its way through the portal circulation, causing hepatofugal flow (ie, flow away from the liver). Backflow typically occurs when the hepatic venous pressure gradient (HVPG) exceeds 12 mm Hg, at which point the backflow starts working its way up the esophageal vein and back down the portal vein. This, in turn, causes the plexus of vessels around the esophagus to swell, leading to the formation of esophageal and gastric junctional varices.

Isolated fundic varices (ie, without junctional or esophageal varices) do not typically occur in the setting of cirrhosis unless some other process is also present. They may occur along with esophageal or junctional varices, but they do not occur in cirrhosis without other sites concurrently involved. To explain how isolated fundic varices could form, we need to posit an obstruction that is proximal to the takeoff of the esophageal vein, causing sinistral, or left-sided, portal hypertension. This is where splenic vein thrombosis comes in. The splenic vein, which joins with the superior mesenteric vein to form the portal vein (see Figure 3-2), runs right along the posterior length of the pancreas. The splenic vein can serve as the bellwether for pancreatic trouble. Splenic vein thrombosis is most common in the setting of either pancreatic cancer or chronic pancreatitis. In both instances, there can be compression and/or stasis of the splenic vein, which leads to secondary thrombosis. When the splenic vein is thrombosed, the blood backs up into the spleen, which in turn becomes swollen and enlarged. This fills the short gastric veins, which connect the spleen with the stomach. This filling, in turn, may lead to isolated fundic varices in the stomach. Since the vascular obstruction is well proximal to the takeoff of the esophageal vein, there is no reason to expect esophageal varices. The history of chronic pancreatitis in this patient raises splenic vein thrombosis as the most likely etiology.

Treatment of gastric varices can be difficult. Unlike esophageal or junctional varices, gastric varices are not easily amenable to endoscopic therapy. Band ligation and sclerotherapy may temporize active bleeding, but they don't seem to hold for long. Cyanoacrylate glue has proven effective but is currently unavailable in the United States and should not be an answer choice on an ABIM Board exam. Intravariceal injection of thrombin has also been reported to be effective, but it too is not standard of care and therefore unlikely to appear on a Board exam. Octreotide can help drop the portal pressure in the acute setting, but it's not a long-term fix for this problem. It would make more sense to fix the underlying problem rather than troubleshoot the varices directly, which are essentially vascular epiphenomena of a more fundamental disorder—in this case, the presumed splenic vein thrombosis from chronic pancreatitis. So that leads us to the ultimate treatment, which is splenectomy. Splenectomy is curative for most patients with isolated fundic varices due to splenic vein thrombosis. If, however, the splenic vein thrombosis is coupled with diffuse thrombosis in the portal and mesenteric veins, then splenectomy would not fix the whole problem.

In cases of severe and recalcitrant bleeding from underlying complex thrombosis involving several vessels, it may be necessary to perform surgery. There are two basic surgical approaches—shunt and nonshunt operations. Surgical shunts come in many types, but the ultimate goal is to decompress the portacaval circulation and relieve the backflow. The splenorenal shunt can work in some cases. If the thrombosis is particularly complex, then nonshunt operations may be necessary. A classic nonshunt operation is the Sugiura procedure, in which the surgeon devascularizes the entire gastroesophageal junction in an effort to take down all the varices. This is rarely performed anymore and is clearly an option of last resort due to the high mortality rate with the surgery itself. Perhaps even more extreme is complete esophageal transection, although this is really directed toward esophageal, not gastric fundic, varices (but worth mentioning for the sake of completeness). Surgical management of bleeding varices remains unusual and mostly limited to centers with considerable experience with these high-risk procedures.

Why Might This Be Tested? Presenting a case of isolated fundic varices is a good way to test your knowledge of vascular anatomy. And since knowing the anatomy has obvious clinical indications, this is a case where remembering your Netter atlas from med school can really come in handy.

Clinical Threshold Alert: If the HVPG exceeds 12 mm Hg, then varices begin to form.

Here's the Point!

Isolated fundic varices in the setting of pancreatitis = Splenic vein thrombosis. Consider splenectomy for treatment.

Vignette 4: Rave

A 20-year-old college student is brought by friends to the emergency department with complaints of nausea, vomiting, and anxiety. He has no significant past medical history, no recent travel, and no unusual food consumption. He denies alcohol use, but his friends mention that he frequently goes to "raves." He is noted to be anxious and diaphoretic in the emergency department with a temperature of 104°F.

On examination, he is jaundiced and has tender hepatomegaly. He is also noted to have jaw-clenching and bruxism (teeth-grinding). A lumbar puncture is performed and is unremarkable. Blood tests reveal the following: INR = 1.5, ALT = 1590, AST = 1440, total bilirubin = 4.2, creatinine = 1.0, WBC = 8.1, hemoglobin = 14.2, platelets = 190, CK = 50, pH = 7.40; blood cultures are pending.

▶ **What is the most likely diagnosis?**

▶ **How can this diagnosis be confirmed?**

Vignette 4: Answer

This is a case of methylenedioxymethamphetamine (MDMA, also known as "ecstasy")-induced hepatotoxicity. If you have a college student presenting with hyperthermia, anxiety, nausea, vomiting, cramping, and muscular rigidity with bruxism and diaphoresis, think of illicit drug use. That seems like a no-brainer, but don't miss it. If the symptoms coincide with acute liver failure, then think of recreational use of ecstasy. The diagnosis can be confirmed with most urine toxicology screening tests.

The pathogenesis of acute MDMA-induced liver injury is multifactorial. Immune mechanisms and reactive metabolites play a role. When combined with hyperthermia, these metabolites can accelerate hepatocellular injury (see Vignette 41 for more on hyperthermia and liver injury). In fact, hyperpyrexia may persist for several hours and patients can become dehydrated, often with complaints of polydipsia. These patients require aggressive cooling, rehydration, and supportive care, and they need to be watched closely for evidence of acute liver failure.

MDMA was first compounded about 100 years ago, but its psychotropic effects were not known until the 1970s when it was used in psychotherapy (until becoming illegal). In the 1980s, MDMA became popular in some nightclub scenes. Soon thereafter, it became—and still is—a common recreational drug in the "rave" culture among adolescents and young adults in the Western world. MDMA is also prevalent on college campuses, where many students hold the misconception that it's a safe drug.

Why Might This Be Tested? MDMA-induced acute liver failure is a well-known problem in young adults using recreational drugs. Public education campaigns are starting to raise better awareness that ecstasy is not a safe drug. Board examiners will expect you to be informed as well.

Here's the Point!

Hyperthermia + Acute hepatitis + College student + Bruxism = Think "ecstasy"

Vignette 5: Right Upper Quadrant Pain in a Young Woman

A 19-year-old college student presents to the student health clinic with a chief complaint of abdominal pain for 3 days, along with progressive fevers and sweats. The pain is constant, sharp, 6 out of 10 in intensity, and located in the right upper quadrant. The pain is worse with deep inspiration and radiates along her right flank and thorax, but not to her right scapula or shoulder. She feels nauseous but has not vomited. She does not report changes in stool frequency or form, has not experienced GI bleeding, and reports no skin rashes or jaundice. Her past medical history is unremarkable, and she does not take medications. She does not report using illicit drugs or herbal preparations. She drinks alcohol socially but reports no intake over the past week. Her last menstrual period was 2 weeks prior to presentation.

On examination, she is febrile with a temperature of 100.9°F. She is not jaundiced and shows no stigmata of chronic liver disease. Her lungs are clear bilaterally. Her abdomen is diffusely tender with voluntary guarding but no rebound tenderness. The abdominal tenderness is most prominent in the right upper quadrant but is also present in the bilateral lower quadrants. Rectal examination reveals brown, heme-negative stool.

She is transferred to the emergency department of the University Hospital, where she undergoes further evaluation with laboratory testing, which reveals the following: WBC = 14 with 92% PMNs, hemoglobin = 13.4, platelets = 212, creatinine = 1.2, AST = 161, ALT = 189, ALP = 56, total bilirubin = 1.3, INR = 1.1, albumin = 3.4, amylase/lipase = normal, beta-HCG = negative, informal bedside right upper quadrant ultrasound is negative.

▶ *What is the next diagnostic step?*
▶ *Why?*

Vignette 5: Answer

This vignette is meant to trick you. If you said the next diagnostic step should be abdominal CT scanning or some other form of diagnostic imaging, then you are wrong. Of course, some kind of imaging may need to be done eventually in this case, but it should not be the very next step.

The correct answer is to perform a pelvic exam. In GI and hepatology we sometimes tend to forget that the pelvis exists, and that can spell trouble—especially in a young woman with abdominal pain. Testing the beta-HCG is a nice start, but that is no substitute for a proper pelvic examination. If you were to perform a pelvic exam on this woman, you would find cervical motion tenderness and adnexal tenderness with bimanual examination. That's because this woman had pelvic inflammatory disease (PID) from *Chlamydia* and has secondary perihepatitis as a consequence of intra-abdominal spread of the infection.

The complex of PID and perihepatitis is also called Fitz-Hugh–Curtis syndrome. Fitz-Hugh–Curtis was first described with gonococcal salpingitis, but it can also occur with Chlamydial infections. The pelvic infection spreads to the abdomen, involves the peritoneal surfaces, and consolidates along the peritoneal reflections in the right upper quadrant around the liver. This gives rise to a purulent, fibrinous exudate around the liver, which looks like so-called violin string adhesions (Board buzzword) on direct visualization. This presents clinically with severe right upper quadrant abdominal pain. In fact, the abdominal pain can become so severe that it dominates the presentation, even though the source of infection is in the pelvis itself. In the case described in this vignette, all eyes were focused on the upper abdomen rather than the pelvis, to the point of bypassing an otherwise vital pelvic examination. The pain can be pleuritic, as seen here. Because it typically involves the anterior surface of the liver, it may not radiate to the shoulder, as seen with biliary colic (although it can radiate to the shoulder). Here the pain radiated around the flank and was worse with breathing—signs of pleurisy. In addition, Fitz-Hugh–Curtis can present with elevated aminotransferase levels in about half of cases.

The bottom line is that in a young woman with right upper quadrant pleuritic pain, fevers, elevated WBC, and elevated liver tests, you need to think about Fitz-Hugh–Curtis and perform a pelvic examination. The CT can wait. In fact, the CT findings in Fitz-Hugh–Curtis are often nonspecific *vis-à-vis* the liver itself, although the pelvic portion of the test should find some changes suggestive of PID. The CT may reveal hepatic capsular enhancement along the anterior surface of the liver in the arterial phase. In any event, a reasonable case can be made for holding on the CT, sparing this young patient the radiation exposure, and instead starting aggressive IV antibiotic therapy for PID as an inpatient while monitoring her carefully for clinical decrements. Would she really escape the emergency room without having a CT performed? Probably not. But don't let that hold you back from performing (or at least recommending, if you are the consulting GI) a pelvic examination.

Why Might This Be Tested? Board examiners want you to think about the entire physical examination, including the pelvic region. Fitz-Hugh–Curtis is a classic diagnosis everyone learns in med school, and including it on the exam provides an opportunity for examiners to see if you have totally forgotten about the pelvis or not. Shooting straight past a pelvic exam can spell trouble;

examiners want to ensure that you are thinking about the pelvic exam as you develop a full differential diagnosis for abdominal pain in women.

Here's the Point!

Sexually active woman + Fever + Pleuritic right upper quadrant pain = Think about Fitz-Hugh-Curtis ... Check pelvic exam

Vignette 6: Polycythemia Vera and Liver Abnormalities

A 46-year-old woman with polycythemia vera presents to the emergency department after awakening to a sense of fullness in her abdomen along with severe right upper quadrant pain. She had neither symptom prior to going to bed. She feels nauseous but has not vomited. There is no diarrhea, melena, or hematochezia. She does not report feeling chills or fever.

On physical examination, she is found to be afebrile, normotensive, slightly tachycardic (heart rate = 106), and tachypneic (respiratory rate = 18) with a normal oxygen saturation of 98% on room air. Her body mass index is 26. She is anicteric but has conjunctival injection. There are extensive excoriations on her skin. Her lungs are clear to auscultation, and her heart is tachycardic but without other arrhythmias. Her abdomen is slightly distended. There is no significant shifting dullness appreciated. The liver edge is tender and palpable 3 cm below the right costal margin and has a total vertical span of roughly 16 cm by percussion. There is voluntary guarding but no rebound tenderness. She has 1+ pitting edema in the bilateral ankles. There are no other significant physical exam findings. Labs include the following: hemoglobin = 18.6, AST = 480, ALT = 302, ALP = 361, total bilirubin = 4.6, albumin = 3.4, creatinine = 1.3.

▶ **What is the most likely diagnosis?**
▶ **How should this be treated?**

Vignette 6: Answer

This is Budd-Chiari syndrome (BCS) secondary to polycythemia rubra vera. BCS is the result of an obstruction to outflow through the hepatic vein (see Figure 3-2) with subsequent hepatic congestion. This manifests with the classic triad of abdominal pain, hepatomegaly, and ascites. A long list of conditions can cause BCS, but all of these conditions have in common an ability to cause venous thrombosis or obstruction. In this case, the patient has polycythemia vera, which is one of the most common underlying conditions to trigger BCS. The polycythemia is not well treated in this case, as evidenced by the conjunctival injection, excoriations, and elevated hemoglobin. Poorly treated polycythemia can lead to hyperviscosity and ultimately hepatic vein thrombosis. Other myeloproliferative disorders, such as essential thrombocythemia and myelofibrosis, are also associated with BCS but at a lower rate than polycythemia vera. Other common associations include pregnancy, medications (including oral contraceptives, in particular), hepatocellular cancer, and a range of prothrombotic conditions such as factor V Leiden mutation and antithrombin III deficiency, among others.

There are some notable epidemiologic characteristics of BCS that might help with Board exam vignettes. In particular, BCS tends to occur in younger patients, with a mean age of presentation of 35 years (although it certainly can be seen in older patients as well, as evidenced in this vignette). BCS is about twice as prevalent in women than men, partly because pregnancy is an important risk factor for BCS. So keep BCS in mind whenever you hear about hepatomegaly and abdominal pain in a pregnant woman, or simply any younger patient, especially when there is concurrent ascites. Remember, you need to know about pregnant women for the Board exam. Test writers seem to love posing questions about pregnant women. We have included several other pregnancy-related vignettes in the pages ahead—stay tuned.

The clinical course of BCS can be variable. In this case the onset was acute; there was not even enough time for ascites to form. Without timely treatment, acute liver failure is possible. In other cases, the syndrome can evolve over months and fly under the clinical radar for a while. In some instances, BCS presents as the initial sign of underlying cirrhosis; in other cases, BCS is discovered in patients with known cirrhosis and refractory ascites only after a fruitless search for other causes of refractory ascites.

Liver tests are usually abnormal in BCS, although the range of liver test abnormalities varies widely. Aminotransferases typically range from around 100 to 600+. Alkaline phosphatase can be in the 200 to 500 range. Total bilirubin can certainly go up, but usually not much beyond 7 to 10 (unless there is acute liver failure).

The injury is most pronounced in zone 3 of the portal lobules. This is a good opportunity to stop and ask yourself why this is so. A review of the anatomy of the portal triads, lobules, and related metabolic zones will provide the answer. So put your first-year med school hat on for a second and take a look at Figure 6-1. This is a stylized version of hepatic acini and portal triads, along with a depiction of the metabolic zones. Yeah, that's right, we made the figure in PowerPoint—it's pretty sweet.

As shown in the figure, the hepatocytes are arranged in roughly hexagonal structures that are bordered by a series of portal triads. The portal triads consist of 3 structures (by definition): the bile ductules, hepatic arterioles, and portal

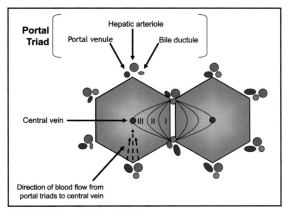

Figure 6-1. Portal circulation and related anatomy.

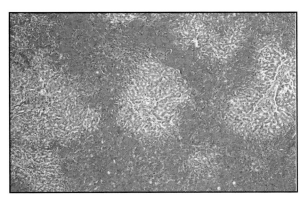

Figure 6-2. Budd-Chiari syndrome with passive congestion in zone 3. (Reprinted with permission of Charles Lassman, MD, UCLA Medical Center.)

venules. The bile ductules form the beginning of the biliary system; they coalesce into the hepatic ducts, which ultimately merge to form the common bile duct. The portal venules receive inflow from the portal vein, and the hepatic arterioles deliver oxygen from the larger hepatic artery. Oxygenated blood from the hepatic arterioles merges with blood from the portal venules. The admixture courses through hepatic sinusoids (not pictured) and collect in the central vein. This anatomic arrangement creates a metabolic gradient comprising zone 1 (periportal zone—maximally oxygenated), zone 2 (intermediate zone), and zone 3 (pericentral zone—minimally oxygenated).

BCS leads to obstructed outflow, so there is backflow and pericentral congestion in zone 3 (Figures 6-1 and 6-2). This makes it even harder for zone 3 to become oxygenated because blood from the triads fights its way upstream against the pressure gradient. When the outflow is acute or severe, zones 1 and 2 become affected as well, which can lead to acute liver failure. In less acute settings, there can still be progressive injury with development of fibrosis within 2 weeks following the initial injury. Left untreated, BCS can progress to bridging fibrosis and, with time, outright cirrhosis. Of note, in BCS there is often a compensatory caudate lobe hypertrophy (Figure 6-3), since flow is not obstructed in this portion due to the accessory hepatic veins that drain directly into the inferior vena cava (IVC). This collateral circulation produces the classic "spider web" appearance on venography. In chronic BCS, the caudate lobe can enlarge enough to cause a secondary IVC obstruction.

Figure 6-3. Budd-Chiari syndrome with characteristic caudate lobe hypertrophy. See text for why this occurs.

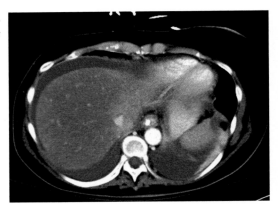

In any event, if you suspect BCS, you should move quickly to clinch the diagnosis. Doppler ultrasound remains a cheap, easy, noninvasive, accurate way to diagnose most cases of BCS. The key is to demonstrate obstructed or attenuated outflow through the hepatic vein. If the study is negative but your pretest likelihood for BCS remains high, then it's reasonable to employ magnetic resonance venography. Computerized tomography does not have a usual role in the diagnosis of BCS. Venography by the interventional radiology service provides the gold standard diagnosis (and can also quantify the pressure measurements) but is cumbersome, expensive, and invasive.

Initial treatment of symptomatic BCS includes anticoagulation, typically with heparin. Longer-term therapy with warfarin is often indicated. If the thrombosis is acute and severe, or if initial anticoagulation is unsuccessful, then catheter-directed thrombolysis may be warranted. Other approaches include transjugular intrahepatic portosystemic shunts (TIPS) and surgical shunts. Liver transplantation may be necessary if there is acute liver failure or if there is secondary cirrhosis in the chronic setting. Of course, it's also crucial to identify the underlying cause of the BCS and, where possible, treat the underlying disorder (in this case, polycythemia vera).

Why Might This Be Tested? First off, as we noted earlier, Board examiners seem to love any question that involves a pregnant patient—a point we will make repeatedly in this book. Although this particular vignette did not feature pregnancy, BCS is an important consideration in a pregnant woman with abdominal pain and a big liver. Second, testing on BCS allows the examiners to check your understanding of vascular anatomy, as with Vignette 3. Third, examiners love figuring out if you can connect common internal medicine diagnoses (in this case, polycythemia vera) with GI and liver conditions. They want to make sure you have not forgotten your basic internal medicine knowledge. And last, they could use this as an opportunity to confirm your knowledge about the microanatomy and metabolic zones of the liver.

Here's the Point!

Ascites + Hepatomegaly + Abdominal pain = Budd-Chiari syndrome (especially in polycythemia vera, pregnancy, and other prothrombotic conditions).

Vignette 7: Can't Get the Mail

A 48-year-old woman with alcoholic cirrhosis complicated by previous variceal hemorrhage now presents with shortness of breath over the past several months. She "can't get the mail anymore" due to marked dyspnea. The dyspnea seems to improve when she lies down. She does not have a previous history of smoking, cardiovascular disease, or lung disease. She has had no chest pain, cough, or fever.

On exam, there are prominent spider angiomas on the upper torso, facial telangiectasias, cyanosis, and clubbing with trace pitting edema in the extremities. Her lungs are clear to auscultation and heart sounds are normal. Lab tests include the following: Na = 138, K = 3.7, creatinine = 1.0, ALT = 38, AST = 46, total bilirubin = 1.0, ALP = 100, albumin = 3.4, INR = 1.2, platelets = 80. An arterial blood gas reveals the following values: pH = 7.47, P_{O2} = 63 mm Hg, P_{CO2} = 34 mm Hg. Pulmonary function tests reveal normal lung volumes but a DL_{CO} of only 50% predicted.

▶ **What is the diagnosis?**

Vignette 7: Answer

This is hepatopulmonary syndrome (HPS). The history and physical exam alone point to the diagnosis even without knowing the results of the other tests. HPS is strongly suggested by the presence of platypnea (improvement in dyspnea when she lies down), coupled with the physical exam findings of clubbing, cyanosis, prominent spider angiomas, and facial telangiectasias. Orthodeoxia (hypoxemia improved when lying down compared with the upright position) can also help you reach the diagnosis.

HPS probably results from the circulation of vasodilators (such as nitrous oxide), leading to intrapulmonary vasodilation. This, in turn, causes hypoxemia by creating a functional A-a gradient from increasing the distance from erythrocytes to the oxygen source as they pass through the lungs. Although 5% to 10% of patients presenting for liver transplant evaluation will have HPS, it seems to be an under-recognized condition. A patient with chronic liver disease or portal hypertension will qualify as having HPS by demonstration of both hypoxemia and intrapulmonary shunting. HPS can be diagnosed when the arterial blood gas reveals a PaO_2 <70 mm Hg and an A-a gradient >20 mm Hg. Of note, a patient with a PaO_2 >80 mm Hg is unlikely to have HPS.

Evidence of intrapulmonary shunting is typically noted with contrast echocardiography with agitated saline. A positive test for HPS results when contrast is seen in the left atrium more than 3 cardiac cycles after the original right ventricular opacification. If the contrast is noted sooner than 3 cardiac cycles, then an intracardiac shunt is likely. Furthermore, the intrapulmonary shunt can be quantified with a technetium macroaggregated albumin (TcMAA) lung perfusion scan to determine uptake in other organs. Under normal conditions, technetium macroaggregates of albumin get trapped in the lung after passing through the right ventricle and do not reach the peripheral circulation. However, with the intrapulmonary shunting of HPS, the macroaggregates can pass into the brain and uptake can be quantified. Thus, a brain uptake of greater than 5% of TcMAA suggests intrapulmonary shunting.

Thus far, medical treatments for HPS have not provided much benefit. However, liver transplantation can reverse the condition in mild to moderate cases. Complete reversal of the intrapulmonary shunting can take up to 1 year, so the effect of liver transplant is not always immediate. Not all patients with HPS do well after liver transplantation, especially those with severe intrapulmonary shunting. The following risk factors can be used to identify HPS patients with severe shunting who may not reverse after liver transplantation: (1) PaO_2 <50 mm Hg (severe hypoxemia); (2) inability to correct hypoxemia with 100% O_2; and (3) TcMAA >40% brain uptake (high shunt fraction).

Why Might This Be Tested? Similar to portopulmonary hypertension (stay tuned for more on that later), the history and physical examination can point to this diagnosis if you understand the pathophysiology. That is why Board examiners love this kind of stuff. Be sure that you don't confuse HPS with portopulmonary hypertension.

Clinical Threshold Alert: PaO_2 must be <70 mm Hg and A-a gradient >20 mm Hg to diagnose HPS. When the PaO_2 falls below 50 mm Hg in HPS, it predicts a poor outcome with liver transplantation. Brain uptake of >5% of TcMAA indicates intrapulmonary shunting in HPS. Liver transplantation is unlikely to be successful when the TcMAA brain uptake exceeds 40%.

Here's the Point!

Liver disease + Hypoxemia + Intrapulmonary vasodilation = Think HPS

Here's the Point!

Consider liver transplantation for HPS with PaO$_2$ 50 to 70 mm Hg

Here's the Point!

Do not consider liver transplantation if TcMAA >40%
(↑ intrapulmonary shunting)

Here's the Point!

Cyanosis and clubbing are common in HPS
(in contrast to portopulmonary hypertension)

Vignette 8: Pregnant Woman With Cirrhosis

A 32-year-old woman is referred to you by her high-risk obstetrician for risk assessment at 13 weeks' gestation. She has well-compensated hepatitis C cirrhosis and has been a nonresponder to therapy in the recent past. She had no significant varices noted on upper endoscopy last year. She feels well and has no symptoms related to liver disease. Her laboratory tests reveal the following: albumin = 3.8, total bilirubin = 1.0, AST = 38, ALT = 25, ALP = 90, creatinine = 0.7, INR = 1.1, WBC = 4.2, hemoglobin = 13.1, platelets = 108, HCV RNA = 800,000 IU/mL. The patient is concerned about transmitting hepatitis C to the baby.

▶ **What test(s), if any, should you order?**

Vignette 8: Answer

This is a tough one, but it highlights several crucial points. First, you should order a Doppler ultrasound of the abdomen to look for a splenic artery aneurysm. There is a 3% to 5% risk of rupture of splenic artery aneurysms in pregnant women with cirrhosis, and a rupture carries up to a 75% maternal mortality rate and a 90% fetal mortality rate. So this can be catastrophic if not identified in advance. Sometimes the initial bleed may be contained in the lesser sac, which leaves time for emergency intervention. Splenic artery aneurysm tends to occur in the third trimester and is multifactorial in etiology. The enlarging uterus can compress the aorta as gestation proceeds, leading to enhanced flow through alterative branches including the splenic artery. Furthermore, the plasma volume is increased in pregnant women with cirrhosis, as is hormone-related weakness of the vasculature. These conditions create a perfect storm for a catastrophe. Thus, if the aneurysm is >2 cm, endovascular or surgical therapy needs to be considered. A question on the Board exam might feature a pregnant woman with cirrhosis presenting with left upper quadrant discomfort, a pulsatile left upper quadrant mass, or a left-sided abdominal bruit (see Vignettes 45 to 49 for more on abdominal bruits in liver disease).

Second, you should also perform an upper endoscopy in this patient. There is a 25% risk of variceal bleeding during pregnancy in women with cirrhosis, and the risk of hemorrhage rises to 75% in pregnant women with large varices. As noted, such hemorrhage could have fatal consequences for both the fetus and the mother. Remember that portal pressures are increased in cirrhosis due to increased plasma volume. For this reason, you should also avoid excessive fluid administration during any admission throughout the pregnancy. Furthermore, there may be increased vascular resistance from external IVC compression by the enlarging uterus. These factors create the greatest risk of variceal hemorrhage in the second trimester and during labor (from the Valsalva maneuver). Therefore, an upper endoscopy should be performed right away in this patient since she is in the second trimester, even though she did not have varices on endoscopy last year. If large varices are found, then action needs to be taken for primary prophylaxis. There are no controlled trials evaluating the safety and efficacy of endoscopic band ligation versus beta-blockade in pregnant patients. Thus, the choice is at the discretion of the treating physicians and is generally made after discussion between the GI and obstetrician. It's worth mentioning that beta-blockers have an FDA pregnancy category C in the first trimester but have a class D rating with risk of intrauterine growth retardation and fetal bradycardia in the second and third trimesters. Specific questions on the direct treatment of varices are unlikely to appear on the exam due to poor consensus of opinion. However, avoidance of labor by caesarean section delivery is recommended to circumvent the elevations of portal pressure and risk of variceal hemorrhage in women with large varices.

Last, you should order a human immunodeficiency virus (HIV) test, especially since the patient wants to know the risk of vertical transmission of hepatitis C. In general, the risk of HCV transmission is quite low (approximately 5%). However, the risk of HCV transmission is increased if there is coinfection with HIV, an elevated HCV RNA level, and/or active intravenous drug use. Transmission rates are not affected by route of delivery. However, there is an increased risk of HCV transmission with use of fetal scalp monitoring or if there is a long duration between membrane rupture and delivery. Breastfeeding does not seem to increase transmission, unless there are cracked, abraded, or bleeding nipples. After delivery, HCV antibody testing should not be checked in newborns of mothers with hepatitis C until well after the first year. Earlier testing can lead to a false-positive diagnosis in the newborn due to transplacental transfer of maternal antibodies. Therefore, HCV RNA should be obtained if needed by the pediatrician in the first year of life.

Why Might This Be Tested? Although many women with cirrhosis are amenorrheic, pregnancy does occur, especially in those with well-compensated disease. Such women can have catastrophic bleeding from a splenic artery aneurysm and/or varices. Prevention is paramount to avoid a disaster. Testing for HCV is now routine during the first obstetrical visit, and positive results will, in turn, lead to consultations for management. You should anticipate that this will be on the exam.

Here's the Point!

Pregnant woman with cirrhosis ⟶ Look for splenic artery aneurysm and varices

Here's the Point!

HCV has a low risk for vertical transmission unless other risk factors are present, including HIV infection, intravenous drug use, or very high HCV viral load.

Vignette 9: Transjugular Intrahepatic Portosystemic Shunt Request

A 58-year-old man with chronic hepatitis C cirrhosis is brought into the emergency department with abdominal distention, malaise, and lethargy. He has required frequent paracentesis for recurrent ascites and has been intolerant to increasing doses of diuretics.

On examination he is icteric with spider nevi, muscle wasting, splenomegaly, hepatic fetor, and tense ascites. Ultrasound shows a shrunken, nodular liver without a mass. His laboratory tests in the emergency department reveal the following: WBC = 5, hemoglobin = 11.5, platelets = 71, bilirubin = 7.2, AST = 96, ALT = 52, ALP = 128, albumin = 2.7, creatinine = 1.5, INR = 1.9, and AFP = 5. The emergency department physician has consulted interventional radiology to evaluate the patient for a Transjugular Intrahepatic Portosystemic Shunt (TIPS) placement. However, the interventional radiologist has asked for your consultation prior to TIPS placement.

▶ **Should this patient receive a TIPS?**

▶ **Why or why not?**

Vignette 9: Answer

This patient has a MELD score equal to 25. A score of 25 means there is about a 25% chance he will die within 3 months without a liver transplant. In someone with this degree of liver dysfunction, placing a TIPS could have disastrous consequences. In patients with poor hepatic synthetic function, TIPS is indicated only when the patient exhibits acute, life-threatening consequences of portal hypertension, such as active variceal hemorrhage. With the advanced degree of liver disease in this patient, there is the added risk of further progression due to portal diversion of blood flow (not to mention all of the other associated TIPS complications, such as encephalopathy, bleeding, sepsis, hemolysis, fistulas, hepatic infarction, hemobilia, and stent dysfunction). The best treatment would include large-volume paracentesis with intravenous albumin in combination with an expedited liver transplant evaluation. TIPS would not be advised in this case unless the patient were in dire straits.

This vignette provides an opportunity to briefly review the MELD scoring system. MELD was initially developed in a multicenter study for patients with cirrhosis undergoing TIPS. It was found to have about an 85% accuracy for predicting death in these patients. After a mandate from the Department of Health and Human Services, MELD replaced the previous Child-Turcotte-Pugh (CTP)-based system. On February 27, 2002, the MELD score was used for liver allocation by the United Network of Organ Sharing (UNOS). I remember being on service when the change occurred. I can just say that it made for quite an interesting day.

The MELD score, which ranges from 6 to 40, has distinct advantages over the CTP system by limiting subjective parameters (such as amount of ascites and encephalopathy) and providing a continuous scale, thereby eliminating the "floor and ceiling" effect that occurred with the CTP system. Of note, INR is the best marker of liver function; therefore, it's the most heavily weighted variable in the MELD scoring system. The predictive value of MELD is independent of common cirrhosis complications, including bacterial peritonitis, variceal hemorrhage, ascites, and encephalopathy. Because these clinical events do not provide an incremental predictive value, MELD is currently calculated with only 3 lab tests (serum INR, total bilirubin, and creatinine) to obtain a score for estimation of 3-month mortality without liver transplantation. At a MELD score of 15 or greater, survival is enhanced 1 year after liver transplant versus remaining on the waiting list. Therefore, most transplant centers designate a MELD score of 15 as the minimal listing score for liver transplantation (although most transplants occur at higher values).

Use of MELD has led to significant improvements in the process of liver transplantation, namely, a reduction in waiting time for transplantation, fewer new patients registered for the waiting list, and the ability to prioritize sicker patients with a greater need for transplantation. Compared to the pre-MELD era, the MELD era has resulted in a diminished mortality rate for those on the transplant list. Post-transplant survival has not decreased, despite transplanting sicker patients. Plus, the use of an evidence-based score makes everyone feel better about making difficult allocation decisions.

However, nothing is perfect. There are some conditions where the MELD score may not accurately predict mortality, and a higher score can be requested through an appeal process to UNOS; such inaccuracy may occur in patients with hepatocellular carcinoma, hepatopulmonary syndrome, and familial amyloidosis, among other conditions. These patients can have progression of disease with a high mortality rate while their MELD score may not necessarily increase in lockstep with their disease severity (which could lead to death while on the list). Furthermore, a subset of patients with a low MELD score have hyponatremia, and these patients may benefit from incorporating serum sodium into the MELD (termed "MELD-Na"). However, the use of diuretics and intravenous fluids can cause marked changes in the serum sodium concentration. Although MELD-Na might be used in the future—as well as some other potential slight revisions of the current MELD scoring system—the core MELD will be the basis for any future prognostication system in the foreseeable future. Therefore, gastroenterologists need to be familiar with applying MELD, and this vignette provides a practical example where the MELD score has implications not only for transplantation but for other decisions as well (in this case, whether to place a TIPS).

Why Might This Be Tested? MELD has replaced the use of the CTP score, which is now considered outdated, for decisions regarding liver transplantation. MELD is being used in other aspects of liver disease, too. So, MELD is here to stay. You simply need to become very familiar with MELD for the exam and for clinical practice.

Clinical Threshold Alerts: A MELD of 15 is the minimal listing score used by most transplant centers. The MELD ranges from 6 to 40 points—this range predicts 3-month survival without liver transplantation in patients with cirrhosis.

Here's the Point!

Avoid TIPS in patients with a high MELD score (25 or more) unless it's a life-threatening emergency or liver transplantation is unlikely.

Vignette 10: Going Vertical

A 25-year-old primigravid Asian woman in her 34th week of pregnancy is referred to you by her obstetrician for management of hepatitis B virus (HBV) infection. The patient was diagnosed with HBV 3 years ago but has steadfastly refused treatment, as she fears long-term side effects of "chemicals." However, she is concerned about passing HBV to her child and wants to know if she should reconsider therapy during the peripartum period. There has been no history of hepatic decompensation. Her pregnancy has been uneventful through 34 weeks of gestation.

Laboratory tests include the following: WBC = 5.5, hemoglobin = 13.1, platelets = 195, ALT = 44, AST = 30, total bilirubin = 1.0, INR = 1.0, albumin = 3.5, creatinine = 0.7, HBeAg = positive, HBeAb = negative, HBV DNA = 4.1 million IU/mL, HBV genotype = C.

▸ **What should you recommend?**

Vignette 10: Answer

The best strategy is to start treatment now with an oral antiviral agent. Then, within 12 hours following delivery, the newborn should receive hepatitis B immunoglobulin (HBIG) and HBV vaccination; this strategy will significantly decrease the risk of vertical transmission of HBV.

This patient is at very high risk for vertically transmitting HBV. The main risk factors include HBeAg positivity and a high viral load (HBV DNA over 1 million IU/mL). With both of these being positive, the patient has a nearly 90% chance of passing HBV to her newborn—a sobering statistic. Transmission usually occurs during delivery. However, caesarean section does not seem to decrease the risk. Treatment with an oral nucleoside/nucleotide analog should be commenced in the third trimester at approximately 34 weeks since delivery typically occurs anytime thereafter. Upon delivery, combining active with passive vaccination in the newborn will further reduce the risk and is about 95% effective. Active vaccination consists of HBV vaccination at delivery and again 1 and 6 months postpartum. Passive vaccination consists of administering HBIG to the newborn at delivery. Of note, HBeAg-negative mothers have a much lower transmission risk (about 20%), but immunoprophylaxis should be given nonetheless to decrease this risk further. Breastfeeding does not bestow an increased risk for HBV transmission.

Several drugs are approved for treatment of HBV infection, including a growing list of nucleoside/nucleotide drugs and pegylated interferon. During pregnancy, where safety is of paramount importance when considering treatment options, interferon would not be advisable due to its side effect profile and pregnancy category C rating. Therefore, a nucleoside or nucleotide analog would be the most appropriate type of therapy to reduce the HBV DNA levels in this patient. You should choose between tenofovir and telbivudine, both of which have an FDA pregnancy category B rating (lamivudine, adefovir, and entecavir are class C). Tenofovir (which has a very low long-term resistance rate) might be favored in this case, since the patient would require long-term therapy given her HBeAg-positive status. However, remember that this patient only wanted to take therapy to decrease her transmission rate. So, if she is not willing to take long-term therapy, then telbivudine (which has an approximate 25% resistance rate at 2 years) would be a reasonable choice to take to the end of pregnancy, since a short course of therapy is unlikely to confer viral resistance. Due to reported exacerbations of liver disease, all HBV-infected women should be closely followed after delivery as well.

While we are on the subject of HBV, here are a few more pearls (this stuff is huge for the Boards, so read carefully!). Along the lines of HBV prophylaxis, keep in mind that chronic HBV patients can acutely "flare" or decompensate when anti-TNF therapy or immunosuppression is administered. Such flares or decompensation occurs up to 50% of the time and can lead to death. On the Board exam, this could be another scenario for linking gastroenterology and hepatology knowledge. For example, the case may involve an HBV carrier with a low DNA level who develops fistulizing Crohn's disease and is planning to start anti-TNF therapy. Regardless of the DNA level, prophylactic therapy with a nucleoside/nucleotide analog should be given during the entire course of anti-TNF or immunosuppressive therapy and should be continued for 6 months after completion.

A similar situation might occur upon titrating prednisone for various conditions. Stay tuned for another vignette on this topic later in this book.

Here's another fact: Acute liver failure from HBV warrants treatment. It was previously thought that treatment may be futile in the setting of acute HBV liver failure. However, data now indicate that timely anti-HBV treatment can improve mortality rates in acute HBV liver failure. Furthermore, even if liver transplant is inevitable, a decreased viral load is important to diminish the risk of post-transplant recurrence. For the same rationale, patients with cirrhosis and any level of viremia require treatment. Both entecavir and tenofovir would be good choices due to their rapid viral suppression and extremely low long-term resistance rates. In fact, treating patients with decompensated HBV cirrhosis can improve hepatic synthetic function. In some instances, patients can have a dramatic response with marked improvement of their MELD score, and the treatment can render them well enough to "de-list" for liver transplantation. So there really is a lot of benefit to treating HBV, even when it might seem like a desperate situation of diminishing returns.

There are currently 8 known genotypes for HBV (genotypes A through H). Of these, 4 predominate in the United States: A, B, C, and D. Genotype A is the most common among African-Americans (remember: *AA has A*) and has the best response to pegylated interferon treatment with up to a 50% e antigen seroconversion rate (as opposed to 30% with the other genotypes). In fact, compared to oral agents, pegylated interferon might be a more effective and cost-effective choice in an HBV genotype A patient with a high ALT and a low viral load. Genotypes B and C are predominantly found among Asians. The patient in this vignette had genotype C, which tends to be a more aggressive form with increased inflammation, rate of progression, and incidence of HCC compared to genotype B (remember: among Asians, genotype B is *better* and C is *crummy*). Genotype D tends to be more commonly found in patients from Eastern Europe and has a generally less favorable prognosis than does genotype A.

Certain subsets of HBV carriers have an increased risk for the development of HCC. In particular, HCC screening should be performed in African Americans over age 20, Asian men over age 40, and Asian women over age 50.

Why Might This Be Tested? There are an estimated 350 million persons worldwide with HBV infection. With increased immigration over the past few decades from endemic regions into the United States, plenty of HBV patients are flying under the radar. They will present in various clinical scenarios (including pregnancy), and you will need to know how to manage them as the treatment is constantly evolving.

Here's the Point!

High HBV DNA + HBeAg-positive $\longrightarrow$ Highest risk for vertical transmission

Here's the Point!

HBV carrier + Anti-TNF therapy ⟶ Use nucleoside/nucleotide analog for prophylaxis (DNA level does not matter)

Here's the Point!

Acute HBV liver failure ⟶ Need to treat with nucleoside/nucleotide analog, even if there is a lack of clinical improvement

Here's the Point!

HBV genotype A (African-Americans) ⟶ Best response to interferon

Here's the Point!

In Asians, HBV genotype B has more indolent disease course than genotype C

Vignette 11: Bubbles

This isn't really a vignette, but take a look at Figure 11-1.

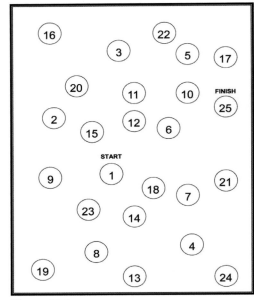

Figure 11.1.

▶ *What is this called?*
▶ *What is it used for?*

Vignette 11: Answer

This is a "trail test," or number connection test (NCT), used to diagnose sub-clinical (aka "minimal") hepatic encephalopathy (HE). Diagnosing and treating overt HE on a timely basis is especially vital. Not only is undiagnosed HE common in patients with otherwise seemingly compensated cirrhosis, but it's also expensive. Overt HE ultimately affects 20% of patients with cirrhosis, requiring more than 55,000 hospitalizations annually and costing over $1 billion per year in health care expenditures. Once HE develops, mortality reaches 35% after 5 years. Surviving patients suffer from diminished health-related quality of life, increased rates of work absenteeism, and decreased work productivity. Patients with HE are also at high risk of motor vehicle accidents and other delirium-related injuries. An additional 50% to 60% of patients with cirrhosis have evidence of subclinical or minimal HE that interferes with cognition and behavior, and one third of these patients ultimately develop overt HE within 2 years of diagnosis. The bottom line is that HE is common and expensive, and you need to know how to diagnose and treat it on a timely basis. You also need to recognize that minimal HE is a legitimate disorder with real-life implications, despite being subclinical or "covert." In fact, there is a fine line between "covert" and overt HE.

Too often we rely on insensitive markers that occur late in the process of HE to make the diagnosis, such as asterixis, hyperreflexia, ataxia, bradykinesia, and overt confusion. By the time someone has, say, asterixis, he or she has already progressed to at least grade 1-2 HE (on the 0 to 4 scale; Table 11-1). Although having asterixis is certainly specific for HE in the setting of cirrhosis, it's by no means sensitive for early disease. We cannot rely on asterixis alone to diagnose HE; we need to do better. Quite frankly, it can be a travesty to evaluate a patient with seemingly compensated cirrhosis, screen for asterixis in the clinic, document "no asterixis" in the chart, confirm a normal serum ammonia level (despite the poor correlation between venous ammonia and clinical symptoms of HE), and then send the patient on his or her way without having diagnosed HE—only to learn that the patient crashed his car into a family crossing the street 3 weeks later. These things do happen. So it's not good enough to write "no asterixis" in the chart and leave it at that. Ruling out asterixis means only that the patient does not have advanced HE yet; it does not rule out earlier HE, which is still potentially deadly—if not for the patient himself, then for the people around him, especially if he drives a car or operates heavy machinery. Diagnosing early HE is serious business.

Screening for signs of HE is worth the time and effort, especially since the effort is relatively small and the benefit is potentially huge. A first step is to ask the patient about sleep, especially variations in sleep-wake cycles. Patients with early HE may develop insomnia at night and hypersomnia during the day, and these diurnal variations may precede the more commonly sought neurologic signs, such as asterixis. Sometimes primary care providers do not recognize this problem and prescribe sleeping pills, which exacerbate the encephalopathy. Patients may also have difficulty concentrating. You can ask this straight up, and many patients will acknowledge that they are having more and more trouble focusing; some describe "brain fog" and other sorts of cloudy thinking. Of course, some patients with HE may not recognize that they are developing forgetfulness or concentration problems, namely because they have HE. So it's

Table 11-1.	
STAGES OF HEPATIC ENCEPHALOPATHY	
Stage	*Description*
0	This is also called minimal hepatic encephalopathy, or MHE. The older term was *subclinical encephalopathy*. These patients exhibit a seemingly normal personality but have minimal changes in their cognitive function, including memory and concentration. This can be picked up with the NCT and other psychometric tests. Otherwise, there are no significant neurologic sequelae.
1	Now things get more involved. These patients have a shorter attention span and reduced ability to perform simple math, like serial 7s. They often have reversal of day-night sleep patterns; diminished awareness and concentration; and signs of irritability, depression, or even euphoria. NCT times get slower. Electroencephalographic (EEG) abnormalities are now detectable. May begin to show asterixis.
2	Now things start getting more serious. Asterixis sets in, and patients experience disorientation, drowsiness, and significant personality changes. These patients can become disoriented and very easily confused. The EEG is clearly abnormal at this point with diffuse slow waves. The patients are hyperreflexic and can exhibit clonus. This is generally obvious to the astute clinician.
3	At this point the patients become sleepy yet arousable. They are totally disoriented regarding time and place. They forget lots of things, have emotional outbursts, and slur their speech. So-called triphasic waves show up on the EEG. If you cannot recognize these clinical features in patients with cirrhosis, then it's time to go back to med school!
4	By stage 4, the patient has basically slipped into a coma. The response to painful stimuli is minimal or nonexistent. If this slips your clinical detection, then it's time to find another line of work.

useful to objectively document evidence of diminished concentration, when present. It's also helpful to elicit history from a family member or spouse who lives with the patient. In the clinic, I like to toss a tennis ball at the patient (gently, of course!) to see if they can catch it, or at least quickly move their hands into position to make the grab. This may also help to make the patient realize that they have HE.

Now let's get back to the image in the vignette. The NCT is a validated technique that can provide objective evidence of HE. The test works by staggering numbers or letters in an arbitrary pattern on a piece of paper, as depicted in Figure 11-1. The patient is asked to link the numbers together as fast as possible by drawing lines between sequential integers. Rather than asking patients to "sequence integers," it's better to use these standardize directions: "On this page you see the numbers from 1 to 25. They have been all scattered about. Your task is to order the numbers by drawing a line between them with a pencil (or pen), starting with the smallest one. You start with the number 1 and draw a straight line from there to 2, then to 3, and so forth. Do this as fast as you can."

A person without HE or other cognitive dysfunction should be able to do this within 30 seconds (try it, it's not that easy to do within 30 seconds but is certainly doable); taking longer suggests HE. Specifically, 31 to 50 seconds tends to correlate with stage 0 to 1 HE, 51 to 80 seconds with stage 1 to 2 HE, and 81 to 120 seconds with stage 2 to 3 HE. Forced termination of the test suggests stage 3. You will not be asked these values on the Board exam, but it's convenient to know them in any event.

If HE is identified, whether overt or minimal, the next step is to consider whether an underlying process might be triggering the HE. There is usually something causing the problem that can be identified and treated. It's not good enough to simply start therapy (more on that shortly) without also considering the underlying cause. Board examiners might want to test this, and we can imagine them developing an HE vignette in which there are clues for an underlying precipitant. Classic examples include overdiuresis from furosemide (leading to a contraction alkalosis, which can precipitate HE); use of sedatives, hypnotics, or opioids; underlying infection (eg, spontaneous bacterial peritonitis); hypoglycemia; gastrointestinal bleeding; electrolyte abnormalities (especially hypokalemia); and a new hepatocellular carcinoma. Be sure to look for these things, both on Board exams and in real life.

Therapy for HE has been difficult and limited in long-term efficacy. In addition to identifying and treating precipitating factors of HE, clinicians traditionally rely on nonabsorbable disaccharides, such as lactulose and lactitol, as the cornerstone of treatment. However, the primary disadvantage of these agents is the high incidence of poorly tolerated adverse events with their use, such as cramping, diarrhea, and flatulence. Moreover, although a Cochrane Systematic Review found that lactulose is more effective than placebo in resolving symptoms of HE, the analysis found no statistically significant difference when limited to studies of high methodological quality. The review concluded that there are insufficient data to support the use of lactulose in the management of HE given the existing data in the literature. However, from clinical experience, it's obvious that lactulose does work in many patients. Taken together, these data indicate that although lactulose may be effective for patients, its effect is not always robust, and compliance is often limited by side effects.

An alternative therapy to nonabsorbable disaccharides is the poorly absorbed oral antibiotic neomycin. Although neomycin has been used in HE for over 3 decades, there are few data to support its efficacy. In fact, no controlled studies have found neomycin to be more effective than standard treatments, and data from one randomized trial found no difference between neomycin and placebo. Moreover, the long-term use of neomycin is limited by nephrotoxicity and ototoxicity, and the incidence of these side effects is even higher in patients with renal insufficiency—a common comorbidity in patients with advanced cirrhosis.

More recently, the minimally absorbed oral antibiotic rifaximin has demonstrated efficacy in maintaining remission of HE. Rifaximin demonstrates high antimicrobial activity against common gut flora in vivo, achieves high gut concentrations, and is negligibly absorbed into the systemic circulation. Randomized controlled trial data reveal that rifaximin is superior to lactulose in the treatment of HE. In addition, rifaximin has lower risks of side effects and better oral tolerability among patients. It was FDA approved for the prevention of recurrence of HE in 2010 after showing a reduced recurrence of overt HE and reduced number of HE-related hospitalizations.

Why Might This Be Tested? HE is prevalent and expensive. Moreover, people with undiagnosed HE can harm themselves and others if not treated in a timely manner. HE has gained increasing attention as a serious disorder with important consequences such as poor driving performance on simulated tests and increased risk for motor vehicle accidents. Thus, it's important to advise patients with HE to avoid driving. Board examiners will want to know that you have heard of minimal HE and that you understand how to identify HE without relying on overt signs like asterixis.

Clinical Threshold Alert: If a patient with cirrhosis takes longer than 30 seconds on an NCT, underlying HE is suggested. This threshold is unlikely to show up on a Board exam, but it's good to have a sense of how to interpret the NCT.

Here's the Point!

Cirrhosis + Sleep trouble + Slow NCT = Hepatic encephalopathy (even if there is no asterixis)

Vignette 12: Fatty Liver Consult

An 18-year-old student without previously known medical problems is referred to you by his family physician for fatty liver on an ultrasound. He saw his family doctor due to persistent mild discomfort in the right upper quadrant after being kicked by a goat at their farmhouse 9 months ago. His mother tells you that his performance at school has also declined in the past 2 years despite tutoring. He was previously a "straight-A student," and now she has trouble reading his small handwriting. His family physician has diagnosed this patient with attention deficit disorder. His mother mentions that she had relatives who "died from liver failure" at a young age. The patient reports no history of alcohol use. His body mass index (BMI) is 21. Laboratory tests reveal the following: total bilirubin = 1.0, albumin = 3.9, ALT = 52, AST = 48, hemoglobin = 12.1, platelets = 160, INR = 1.0, iron saturation = 20%.

▶ **What is the diagnosis?**

▶ **What test(s) could you order to confirm the diagnosis?**

▶ **What else should you tell the patient to decrease the risk of progression?**

Vignette 12: Answer

This is Wilson disease (WD), or hepatolenticular degeneration. WD was described by Kinnear Wilson about 100 years ago. It's an autosomal recessive condition marked by impaired biliary secretion of copper as a result of a mutation in the ATP7B WD gene on chromosome 13; this leads to accumulation of copper in the liver with resulting injury, almost always occurring before 30 years of age. As excess copper is released into the bloodstream, it's deposited into other organs such as the brain, cornea, and kidneys. In the kidneys the copper typically deposits in the renal tubular cells, which leads to a form of Fanconi syndrome. Of note, the ATP7B is the same gene responsible for the copper-deficient state found in Menkes disease, which leads to growth failure, coarse and sparse hair, and a deterioration of the nervous system. Menkes disease is found in early childhood. Therefore, you will not see Menkes disease on the exam, but you can use this knowledge to impress your colleagues!

Patients with WD may also present with neuropsychiatric symptoms. Micrographia (as seen in this case) is a classic symptom of WD and can also be seen in Parkinson's disease. In fact, WD can present with other Parkinsonian symptoms, including the tremor, drooling, rigidity, and risus sardonicus, or uncontrollable grinning. Patients with neurologic symptoms tend to present at a younger age and may show a decline in school performance that can be misconstrued as attention deficit disorder.

Fatty liver is commonly seen in WD, and the patient can be misdiagnosed as having nonalcoholic steatohepatitis (NASH). However, this patient had a normal BMI and did not have other significant medical history, which undermines the diagnosis of NASH. In fact, there is quite a bit of histologic and clinical variation in WD. Histologically, patients can present with interface hepatitis similar to autoimmune hepatitis. So, if a young patient is not responding to steroids for autoimmune hepatitis, think of WD as a distinct possibility. Patients with WD can also present with acute liver failure, which is usually accompanied by hemolytic anemia due to the excess free copper in the circulation and a markedly low serum ALP (less than 40 IU/L).

Serum ceruloplasmin is the first test that should be ordered. A low level (less than 20 mg/dL) is considered positive, but further testing is needed for confirmation of the diagnosis. A very low level (less than 5 mg/dL) can clinch the diagnosis with the right clinical picture. A 24-hour urine copper level should be checked, and the diagnosis is confirmed when the copper level is more than 100 mcg. Alternatively (or as an adjunct test), you might order a slit-lamp examination for Kayser-Fleischer (KF) rings. The greenish-brown color of these rings is due to copper deposited in a granular complex with sulfur in Descemet's membrane of the cornea. KF rings are not pathognomonic for WD (they can also be found in other chronic cholestatic conditions such as primary biliary cirrhosis). KF rings are present in about half of WD patients with solely hepatic manifestations; however, they are present in at least 90% of cases with neurologic involvement (such as in this case). Of note, the sunflower cataract (copper deposits in the lens) is another ocular manifestation of WD. A liver biopsy can also be helpful; a hepatic copper concentration of 250 mcg/g dry weight can seal the diagnosis (Figure 12-1). However, as with KF rings, other chronic cholestatic diseases can also cause an elevation in the hepatic copper concentration.

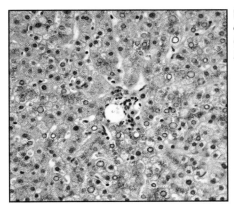

Figure 12-1. Rhodanine stain of the liver in Wilson disease. Red granules of copper are seen in the hepatocytes. (Reprinted with permission of Charles Lassman, MD, UCLA Medical Center.)

Treatment for WD is lifelong and consists of using a metal chelating agent such as trientine or penicillamine to remove accumulated copper. Zinc can also be used to prevent future reaccumulation and to maintain clinical remission (zinc interferes with GI absorption of copper). Twenty-four-hour urinary copper levels can be followed to assess response and compliance to therapy. Response to therapy is usually excellent, provided the patient is diagnosed before the onset of decompensated cirrhosis or acute liver failure. However, neuropsychiatric manifestations may not resolve completely. Liver transplantation provides a cure for the liver disease since it corrects the metabolic defect in the liver. Thus, patients who undergo liver transplantation do not need chelation or zinc therapy.

Foods that contain a large amount of copper should be avoided to minimize further copper accumulation. These include chocolate, nuts, organ meats (especially liver—perhaps that is a little too obvious), shellfish, and mushrooms. The patient in this vignette lives on a farm and likely is drinking well water, which may be entering the house through copper pipes. The home's water supply will need to be checked for copper content. If it's elevated, then the family should find other forms of portable water or else invest in a home water purification system. Also, the family should be mindful to avoid cooking or storing food or water in copper containers or cookware.

Why Might This Be Tested? WD is an uncommon disease with plenty of extrahepatic manifestations and unique diagnostic values, making it a favorite of the examiners. You just have to know this stuff. For that reason we will reinforce some of this information later on in this book.

Clinical Threshold Alerts: The following values all suggest the diagnosis of WD:
1. Serum ceruloplasmin <20 mg/dL
2. 24-hour urinary copper excretion >100 mcg
3. Hepatic copper concentration >250 mcg/g dry weight
4. Serum ALP level <40 IU/L in acute liver failure

Here's the Point!

Neurologic symptoms with liver disease in a young patient =
Think Wilson Disease

Vignette 13: Screening for Varices in Cirrhosis

A 48-year-old man with compensated cirrhosis from chronic hepatitis C is referred for consideration of screening for esophageal varices. The patient has not previously received an upper endoscopy. He has a MELD score of 14; meets criteria for Child classification A disease; and has not developed variceal bleeding, encephalopathy, or ascites.

On physical examination, his heart rate is 86, blood pressure 142/86, respiratory rate 14, and temperature 98.8°F. He is found to have minimal but present scleral icterus, spider angiomas on the anterior chest, a firm liver edge 2 cm below the right costal margin, a palpable spleen tip, and 1+ pitting edema at the ankles. There is no abdominal distention, shifting dullness, or caput medusae. There is no asterixis, and the patient readily passes office-based psychometric testing with a trail test, cube reproduction test, and serial 7s.

Laboratory testing reveals the following: hemoglobin = 12.2, WBC = 3.4, platelets = 72, INR = 1.2, total bilirubin = 2.4, creatinine = 1.3, albumin = 3.1, AST = 38, ALT = 56, ALP = 47, AFP = 8. Right upper quadrant ultrasonography reveals a nodular-appearing liver with a portal vein diameter of 2 cm and a portal vein thrombus.

▶ *What specific features raise the risk of underlying varices, other than having cirrhosis itself?*

▶ *Do guidelines recommend screening for varices in this situation?*

Vignette 13: Answer

Up to one-half of patients with compensated cirrhosis have moderate or large underlying esophageal varices. Once esophageal varices form, the risk of variceal bleeding within 2 years is 20% to 35%, and the risk of dying from an initial variceal bleed is around 20% (historically as high as 50%). In light of the substantial human and economic costs of variceal hemorrhage, several strategies have been developed for primary prophylaxis against an initial bleed, including beta-blocker therapy, combination beta-blocker and nitrate therapy, and endoscopic band ligation.

However, the clinician evaluating a patient with compensated cirrhosis is often unaware of whether there are underlying varices and is faced with the dilemma of whether or not to perform screening upper endoscopy. Proponents of screening endoscopy contend that the procedure allows for the detection of esophageal varices, targeted endoscopic treatment in patients with esophageal varices, and reduction of unnecessary therapy in patients without esophageal varices. The American College of Gastroenterology (ACG) and the American Association for the Study of Liver Diseases (AASLD) recommend universal screening endoscopy in patients with compensated cirrhosis, followed by active therapy for those patients with esophageal varices. Opponents argue that a strategy of universal screening endoscopy requires an excessive use of resources to identify the subset of at-risk patients, and that empiric medical therapy may be a more cost-effective approach that can be carried out in the primary care setting, without reliance on specialist care.

In deference to both strategies, another approach is to perform screening endoscopy only in patients at high risk for underlying esophageal varices. Several studies have identified 4 clinical variables that significantly correlate with the presence of varices including platelet count <88,000/mL, elevated INR, splenomegaly, and portal vein diameter >13 mm on ultrasonography. Each of these predictors is independently associated with underlying varices. Of note, the presence of ascites, encephalopathy, and level of bilirubin elevation have not been found to be independently predictive of varices. The patient in this vignette has thrombocytopenia and portal vein dilatation, both of which indicate an elevated HVPG and therefore a higher-than-average risk of varices. These clinical predictors may allow physicians to select the subgroup of patients with cirrhosis who are most likely to have underlying varices and therefore are most likely to benefit from screening endoscopy. But it turns out that the cost-effectiveness of screening endoscopy does not get any better if we use these rules; they are good to know about, but in the end, the guidelines basically recommend screening for varices in all patients with compensated cirrhosis, not just those with a low platelet count, big portal vein, splenomegaly, and elevated INR.

In passing, it's worth reviewing the role of HVPG monitoring in cirrhosis. Data indicate that variceal formation increases once the HVPG exceeds 12 mm Hg. Furthermore, the higher the HVPG, the higher the portal pressure and higher the risk of variceal bleeding. The goal of beta-blocker therapy is to drop the HVPG below 12 mm Hg. Of course, that does not happen in many people on beta-blocker therapy, even if they are compliant. The failure of beta-blocker therapy to drop the HVPG below 12 mm Hg partly explains why the risk reduction for variceal hemorrhage is only around 50% with beta-blockers (which isn't bad, but isn't great either). In contrast, prophylactic endoscopic band ligation drops the risk of bleeding by up to two-thirds and can work even if the HVPG remains above 12 mm Hg. In general, HVPG monitoring is invasive, expensive, and not routinely performed in the United States. Some argue that it's most useful in patients on the waiting list for a transplant in order to maximize therapy. In fact, it has been shown that routine HVPG monitoring is cost-effective in this high-risk group awaiting transplantation. But otherwise, guidelines do not recommend routine HVPG testing in patients with cirrhosis, even if they have varices. The surrogate markers for beta-blocker therapy are to monitor blood pressure and heart rate with a goal to drop the heart rate to 55 to 60 beats per minute and to drop the systolic blood pressure by 25% as tolerated. Patients who cannot meet those goals despite compliance with therapy should be moved to another approach, such as endoscopic band ligation.

It's also worth taking a moment to review how to manage (or not manage, as the case may be) portal vein thrombosis. Here's the deal: Portal vein thrombosis is quite common in cirrhosis. Its presence confirms hepatofugal flow and high portal pressures. It's typically an epiphenomenon of underlying portal hypertension, not a disease unto itself in need of active therapy. Heparin is generally not indicated for portal vein thrombosis in the setting of cirrhosis, unless there is extensive thrombosis that could preclude liver transplantation. Follow-up imaging is recommended to ensure stability of the thrombus and to exclude hepatocellular carcinoma. More importantly, you should focus on the basic principles of cirrhosis care, which are described throughout this book. Stay tuned for another vignette on this topic that tells the tragic story of unnecessarily treating a portal vein thrombus.

Why Might This Be Tested? Varices are common, so you should know about their basic management principles. This vignette contains several important and highly testable points about variceal screening and management. First, remember that current guidelines recommend routine screening for varices in basically all cirrhotics, whether you agree with that or not. Second, remember that you can determine whether patients are at higher-than-average risk for varices using readily available clinical data. Third, remember that the point of beta-blocker therapy is to drop the HVPG below 12 mm Hg—a clinical threshold that might be useful to know on the Board exam. Fourth, remember that beta-blocker therapy should drop a patient's heart rate to 55 to 60 and systolic blood pressure by 25%; these are surrogate markers for a decrease in HVPG. And finally, don't go nuts when you see a portal vein thrombus in a patient with cirrhosis—it's usually a sign of high portal pressures, but not a disease unto itself. All of these facts are eminently testable.

Clinical Threshold Alert: If the HVPG exceeds 12 mm Hg, then the risk of underlying varices goes up significantly; the goal of beta-blocker therapy is to drop the HVPG below this level. Clinical surrogate markers of diminished portal pressure include a heart rate of 55 to 60 and a systolic blood pressure drop of 25% upon initiation of beta-blocker therapy. While this is admittedly redundant of what has just been said, it bears repeating, and these thresholds are well worth memorizing. In addition, when the portal vein diameter exceeds 13 mm on ultrasonography or when the platelet count falls below 88,000, the risk of varices rises independent of other clinical factors.

Here's the Point!

Independent predictors of underlying varices in cirrhosis:
- Portal vein diameter >13 mm
- Splenomegaly
- Platelet count <88,000
- Elevated INR

Vignettes 14 to 22: DILI Delight

It seems like virtually every medication and herbal supplement can affect the liver. Obviously that is an exaggeration, but there is a definitely a core set of medications and herbals that are especially known for causing drug-induced liver injury, or DILI. You can bet that DILI will show up on the exam; DILI is big time, and it's something we're always dealing with. For that reason, we have prepared a series of mini-vignettes that feature classic DILI scenarios. For each question, identify the culprit medication or herbal, and specify the related adverse event described in the scenario.

14. A woman began using a dietary supplement touted for its weight loss benefits and for relieving menopausal symptoms. After beginning to use the supplement, she became jaundiced and rapidly encephalopathic. Liver biopsy revealed hepatic necrosis. She subsequently required liver transplantation.

15. A patient is found to have liver test abnormalities 2 months after beginning an antiarrhythmic for atrial fibrillation. Relevant labs include the following: AST = 52, ALT = 86, ALP = 110, total bilirubin = 1.4, INR = 1.0, albumin = 3.4. Liver biopsy reveals phospholipid-laden lysosomal lamellar bodies.

16. A patient is treated with an antibiotic for a urinary tract infection (UTI). She develops icterus. Liver tests reveal AST = 35, ALT = 59, ALP = 620, total bilirubin = 2.6, INR = 1.1, albumin = 3.5.

17. A gymnast begins taking an anti-inflammatory medication for musculoskeletal pain. Eight weeks later she is found to have an elevated liver test as part of a routine physical examination. She has the following liver test values: AST = 225, ALT = 280, ALP = 109, total bilirubin = 1.9, INR = 1.3, albumin = 3.4. **Hint:** What commonly prescribed anti-inflammatory received an FDA warning for this in 2009?

18. A patient with inflammatory bowel disease (IBD) begins to take a steroid-sparing agent. Routine liver testing 4 weeks later reveals an elevated AST and ALT. The patient is otherwise asymptomatic.

19. A patient with ulcerative colitis begins to take a steroid-sparing agent. Four weeks later he is hospitalized with ascites, marked weight gain, and right upper quadrant abdominal pain. He is found to have an enlarged and tender liver on examination, and laboratory tests reveal hyperbilirubinemia (total bilirubin = 4.2) and thrombocytopenia (platelets = 105).

20. A bodybuilder develops jaundice. Physical examination reveals an enlarged liver. Labs include ALP = 462, GGT = 387, AST = 82, ALT = 90, total bilirubin = 1.8.

21. A health freak develops elevated liver tests and is found to have lipid-filled stellate cells on liver biopsy.

22. A patient with metabolic syndrome is prescribed a statin. The aminotransaminases elevate to twice the upper limit of normal, and the patient's primary care physician sends the patient to you for management. The patient is otherwise asymptomatic. Should you stop the statin?

Vignettes 14 to 22: Answers

14. This is severe liver injury from kava kava, a botanical product obtained from the roots of the *Piper methysticum* shrub indigenous to the South Pacific. Although knowing about the arcane *Piper methysticum* bush will provide you with nothing more than championship-level minutiae, recognizing kava kava and understanding its risks can be vital information. Kava kava is an herbal dietary supplement that has been used throughout the world for several indications, including anxiety, sleep disturbances, weight loss, and menopausal symptoms. It may have an appealing name, but what it can do to the liver is not appealing—in fact, it can be downright deadly. There are hundreds of case reports of severe hepatotoxicity related to kava kava; in some of these patients, the hepatotoxicity led to acute liver failure resulting in transplantation and/or death. The hepatotoxic effect of kava kava is unpredictable. In case series, the time to adverse event varied dramatically, ranging from just a few weeks to several years following initiation of the supplement. It remains unknown exactly how kava kava causes liver damage. The histologic pattern of injury is also somewhat variable and includes hepatic necrosis, lobular hepatitis, and a cholestatic pattern.

Because of the severe injury related to kava kava, the FDA issued a consumer warning in 2002 regarding its hepatotoxicity. The FDA advises special caution in patients who have pre-existing liver disease and further recommends that "health-care providers should consider questioning patients with evidence of hepatic injury about the use of dietary supplements and herbal products" in general. While it may seem obvious to ask about herbals, all too frequently health-care providers neglect to do this. If you don't ask about herbals, it's time to start. Make it routine. You can save lives by advising patients to stop potentially hepatotoxic agents if you catch it early enough. So the next time you have a patient with elevated aminotransferase levels, be sure to ask about herbal supplements as part of the usual workup.

Some traditional Chinese herbal supplements, in particular, are known to cause liver test abnormalities or even acute liver failure. However, because these supplements are often a blend of many agents, it can be difficult to pinpoint the culprit. For that reason, take caution whenever a patient is taking unnamed or blended herbal supplements, especially when he or she has evidence of liver test abnormalities. A full accounting of all the known herbals and botanicals associated with liver injury is outside the scope of this little review, but other culprits include ma huang (Ephedra), mistletoe, alkaloid-containing herbal teas, germander blossoms (used for abdominal pain, by the way), and chaparral, among many others.

Here's the Point!

> Liver test abnormalities + Any herbal = Suspect the herbal until proven otherwise
>
> Think about kava kava, ma huang (Ephedra), mistletoe, alkaloid-containing teas, germander, and chaparral, among many others.

15. This is amiodarone toxicity. When a patient presents with heart arrhythmias and liver test abnormalities, think about amiodarone along with whatever else might be on your mind (eg, right heart failure, hemochromatosis with cardiomyopathy). Amiodarone can be an effective antiarrhythmic, but it's also known to cause liver injury. Case series indicate that roughly 1 in 4 patients develop asymptomatic elevations in liver enzymes after starting amiodarone, and guidelines suggest discontinuing amiodarone if the liver test values double early in the therapeutic course. Clinically significant liver injury is less frequent but still occurs in a fair number of patients—roughly 3% develop hepatitis. Long-term amiodarone therapy can lead to chronic liver injury in a smaller group of patients, with cirrhosis and liver failure described after cumulative doses begin to mount (although there is no magical cumulative dose beyond which liver injury is definitely known to occur). Because long-term amiodarone therapy increases the risk of chronic liver injury, guidelines suggest using the lowest dose of amiodarone possible and monitoring liver tests both at baseline and at 6-month intervals. Interestingly, amiodarone-induced liver injury is marked by Mallory bodies along with steatosis, phospholipidosis, intralobular inflammation, and—when advanced—fibrosis. A great Board buzzword is "phospholipid-laden lysosomal lamellar bodies," which can be found on electron microscopy in amiodarone-induced liver injury. Because other conditions are also associated with Mallory bodies (see Vignettes 34 to 37 for details), not the least of which is alcohol-induced liver injury, some have suggested testing for phospholipidosis to help distinguish amiodarone from alcohol in the arrhythmic alcoholic on amiodarone (the "triple A") with liver test abnormalities. Bear in mind, however, that amiodarone is not alone in causing phospholipidosis; other culprits include amitriptyline, chloroquine, chlorpromazine, and thioridazine, among others.

Here's the Point!

> **Arrhythmias + Liver test abnormalities + Phospholipid-laden lysosomal lamellar bodies = Amiodarone toxicity**

16. This is most likely cholestasis from trimethoprim-sulfamethoxazole (TMP-SMX). TMP-SMX can cause an acute cholestatic injury, typically seen biochemically with an ALP greater than twice the upper limit of normal or an ALT/ALP ratio of <2. This is in contrast to acute hepatocellular injury, in which the ALT is at least twice the upper limit of normal and the ALT/ALP ratio is >5. Drug-induced cholestasis is traditionally divided into the "bland" type of pure canalicular injury, in which there is primarily an elevated ALP out of proportion to the liver enzymes, and so-called hepatocanalicular injury, in which the liver enzymes are elevated along with the ALP. The latter injury can be more serious than the pure canalicular pattern, since it often involves hepatocyte necrosis and destructive cholangitis. Another commonly used antibiotic, erythromycin, is especially known to cause the mixed hepatocanalicular pattern. But erythromycin is not commonly employed for the treatment of urinary tract infections, making it less likely to be the culprit in this particular case. However, if you see a patient with gastroparesis who is now developing cholestasis, you might consider erythromycin, which is sometimes used as a prokinetic. Amoxicillin-clavulanate and tetracycline are also known to cause cholestatic injury, including the mixed hepatocanalicular pattern. You might have thought about nitrofurantoin, which is indeed used for urinary tract infections and is also known to cause liver injury. However, nitrofurantoin is most commonly associated with a hepatocellular injury marked by elevations in the AST and ALT, and with an autoimmune-type of chronic hepatotoxicity; it's less commonly associated with an acute cholestatic injury pattern.

Here's the Point!

UTI + Cholestasis = Think TMP-SMX
URI + Cholestasis = Think amoxicillin-clavulanate
Gastroparesis + Cholestasis = Think erythromycin

17. This is most likely acute hepatocellular injury from diclofenac. Diclofenac is a nonselective nonsteroidal anti-inflammatory drug (NSAID) that is known to cause liver injury. In fact, the relationship between diclofenac and liver injury is strong enough for the FDA to have issued a public warning in December 2009 regarding cases of diclofenac-induced hepatotoxicity. There have been instances of diclofenac causing acute liver failure requiring transplantation or leading to death. For some reason the relationship between diclofenac use and liver injury seems stronger in women than in men. The FDA suggests that providers monitor liver enzymes "periodically" in patients receiving long-term diclofenac therapy, and definitely monitor liver enzymes within the first 4 to 8 weeks of therapy.

The acute liver injury caused by diclofenac can be idiosyncratic; it's hard to predict when, and in whom, it will occur. But acute liver failure is thankfully rare (the true incidence is not clear, since it's hard to know the exposed denominator). Asymptomatic liver enzyme elevations greater than 3 times the upper limit of normal are more common and better described, occurring in around 1% to 4% of patients receiving diclofenac.

It's notable that diclofenac is also associated with an autoimmune-type chronic hepatitis in addition to the acute hepatotoxicity-type injury. This form of chronic liver injury is similar to the type I, or classic, form of autoimmune hepatitis. The histologic appearance is also similar to autoimmune hepatitis, and patients with diclofenac-induced autoimmune hepatitis are also more likely to have underlying autoimmunity, including antinuclear antibody (ANA) positivity or the presence of smooth muscle antibodies. As an aside, other drugs associated with the autoimmune-type of hepatotoxicity include methyldopa, minocycline, nitrofurantoin (see Vignette 16), phenytoin, and propylthiouracil, among others.

By the way, if you were thinking about acetaminophen when you read the vignette, you were wrong—acetaminophen is not an anti-inflammatory, and warnings about its liver toxicity were issued way before 2009. But more on acetaminophen-induced liver damage in Vignette 27.

Here's the Point!

NSAID use + Liver trouble = Think diclofenac

Here's the Point!

Autoimmune-type chronic liver injury from medications, think:
- **Diclofenac**
- **Minocycline**
- **Nitrofurantoin**
- **Phenytoin**
- **Propylthiouracil**

18. This is hepatocellular injury from azathioprine (AZA) or 6-mercaptopurine (6-MP). For a full explanation of the metabolic by-products and associated adverse events of AZA/6-MP, refer to the first *Acing* book; there we provide a detailed account of how AZA/6-MP is metabolized and how to interpret variations in the levels of its by-products. In short, AZA is nonenzymatically converted into 6-MP. This, in turn, can be broken down into several by-products, one of which is 6-methylmercaptopurine (6-MMP), an inactive metabolite that can cause hepatotoxicity. The breakdown of 6-MP to 6-MMP is catalyzed by the enzyme thiopurine methyltransferase (TPMT). This enzyme is important because genetic variations in TPMT have big implications in AZA/6-MP dosing and toxicity. Ninety percent of the population has high TPMT enzyme activity, in which there is a higher production of 6-MMP and lower production of the 6-thioguanine nucleotides (6-TGN). Some of these patients can potentially have hepatotoxicity with doses of AZA/6-MP that would normally be therapeutic. Levels of 6-MMP above 5700 can be associated with liver toxicity and should be avoided. However, they would be less likely to have bone marrow toxicity and myelosuppression due to the lower 6-TGN.

Here's the Point!

Patient with IBD bumps liver enzymes after starting AZA/6-MP = Think about high TPMT enzyme activity versus supratherapeutic dosing

19. This is veno-occlusive disease (VOD), also known as sinusoidal obstruction syndrome (SOS), from AZA. So AZA strikes again. VOD is marked by a non-thrombotic obstruction of the central hepatic venules with resulting sinusoidal dilation and congestion throughout the liver. It's caused by a diffuse endothelial injury of unclear etiology. Although the exact pathogenesis remains unclear, risk factors for VOD are well recognized. AZA is a classic culprit, although the absolute risk of developing VOD from AZA is exceedingly small, especially when AZA is used in inflammatory bowel disease (there are case reports, but they are very rare). Other more common culprits include bone marrow transplantation, in which VOD complicates up to 50% of cases, and various forms of chemotherapy (especially busulfan and cyclophosphamide) and Jamaican herbal teas. Clinically, patients with VOD typically have a conjugated hyperbilirubinemia >2 mg/dL, ascites, painful hepatomegaly, and marked weight gain over a short period. Thrombocytopenia may occur as well. Liver biopsy is not necessary to make the diagnosis, but when it's performed (usually through a transjugular approach given the thrombocytopenia), it reveals widening of the subendothelium in the central venules and sinusoidal congestion. Whereas treatment for VOD is very difficult in the setting of bone marrow transplant, case reports of AZA-induced VOD often reveal biochemical and symptomatic resolution following discontinuation of the offending agent.

Here's the Point!

Patient with IBD gets painful hepatomegaly and has high bilirubin level after starting AZA = Think about rare but serious veno-occlusive disease

20. This is peliosis hepatis from anabolic steroids. Peliosis hepatis is a rare liver disorder marked by multiple blood-filled cystic spaces throughout the liver parenchyma (not to be confused with VOD, as described in Vignette 19). The cysts of peliosis hepatis do not have an endothelial lining but instead communicate directly with the hepatic sinusoidal system. Peliosis is associated with a range of conditions, including HIV, where it's most commonly a consequence of *Bartonella* infection, but it can also be found in nonimmunosuppressed patients.

Peliosis has been described in users of anabolic steroids, as well users of azathioprine (there it is again), oral contraceptives, vitamin A, and hydroxyurea, among many other medications. Rather than memorize this tedious list, you should focus on remembering anabolic steroids and HIV as the most common and most important associations. Peliosis usually presents with fever, weight loss, and jaundice in the setting of an enlarged liver. Because peliosis involves cystic lesions in the liver, the ALP and GGT are elevated and out of proportion to the AST and ALT (which are elevated to a lesser degree). The bilirubin is characteristically normal or near normal. CT scans will show an enlarged and heterogeneous liver, and may also reveal a large spleen and abdominal lymphadenopathy. Treatment is to remove the culprit agent. However, when peliosis occurs in the setting of acquired immunodeficiency syndrome (AIDS), you should treat with erythromycin 2 g daily (which hopefully will not cause a cholestatic hepatocanalicular injury) to empirically cover *Bartonella* infection.

Here's the Point!

AIDS + Elevated ALP/GGT + Fever + Weight loss + Enlarged liver + Bartonella = Peliosis hepatis

21. This is hypervitaminosis A. Vitamin A (retinoic acid) can be a good thing, but too much of a good thing can cause problems. There are high concentrations of vitamin A in certain foods, including liver, kidney, and egg yolks. Beta-carotene, in contrast, is a pro-vitamin A substance. Whereas vitamin A is found in animal products, beta-carotene is usually found in green, leafy vegetables. Another important difference is that vitamin A can cause direct liver injury, whereas beta-carotene does not—it needs to be converted to vitamin A before wreaking havoc. So it's less common to develop liver injury from beta-carotene overdose than from vitamin A overdose. Most commonly, however, hypervitaminosis A occurs from taking too much retinoic acid supplementation. This is especially common among "health nuts" who view vitamin A as an important part of their overall health and well-being. Vitamin A can cause proliferation of the stellate cells with lipid infiltration and, over time, is even associated with cirrhosis and veno-occlusive disease.

Here's the Point!

Health freak + Lipid-filled stellate cells = Vitamin A toxicity

22. No, you should not stop the statin. This mini-vignette provides an excuse to review the hepatotoxicity (or lack thereof) of statin therapy. There is no question that statins are associated with liver test abnormalities, but that does not mean that statins are dangerous or need to be stopped at the earliest sign of liver trouble. Around 10% of statin users will have mild elevations in their ALT levels. Usually these elevations are pretty minimal, although in up to 1% to 3% of users the elevations exceed 3 times the upper limit of normal (ULN). However, some large, randomized controlled trials of statin versus placebo have found virtually no difference in the prevalence of elevated ALT between statin and placebo. One study evaluated lovastatin versus placebo in over 6500 subjects in a 5-year follow-up study and found that ALT elevations exceeding 3 times ULN were virtually the same between the lovastatin (0.6%) and placebo (0.3%) groups. Similarly, multiple studies in thousands of patients have found no difference in ALT levels between patients using simvastatin versus placebo. The same thing has been found with pravastatin and atorvastatin. Fluvastatin may have a slightly higher risk than placebo, but even there the risk is small.

You get the point—statins probably don't do much to the liver (if anything), and they end up getting a bad rap. Yet gastroenterologists and hepatologists are bombarded by consults asking them to comment on or manage the risk of statin-induced hepatotoxicity. Hepatologists, in particular, usually wrinkle their brows at the consult and mumble something about statin-induced hepatotoxicity being overblown. In fact, a recent review of the topic in the *American Journal of Gastroenterology* by T. Bader started like this: "Statin-induced hepatotoxicity is a myth. 'Myth' is used here to mean a false collective belief that, despite factual contradiction, endures as suspicion." Bader went on to emphasize that the "elevation of serum ALT is not a disease. At worst, the ephemeral out-of-range ALT values represent adaptation to exposure to statins by the different organs involved in ALT regulation. In the liver this is done by alteration of metabolic enzyme and transporter systems to process the drug. When a statin is continued, despite elevations of ALT, the ALT eventually returns to normal unless some other cause for liver disease exists." Notably, transient ALT elevations have also been observed in other classes of anticholesterol agents, suggesting that transient rises may actually reflect that the drug is working and that the elevation is, in fact, the result of an agent lowering cholesterol, not a direct cause of parenchymal damage. In fact, statins are being studied by hepatologists in the setting of nonalcoholic fatty liver disease (NAFLD) as a therapeutic approach to managing the metabolic syndrome. So, if liver docs are comfortable using a statin even in the setting of liver disease, internists should probably be comfortable using the drug in settings without liver disease, even if there is a transient minor rise in aminotransferase levels. Perhaps surprisingly, there are even data that the efficacy of anti-HCV therapy is enhanced in the setting of statin therapy, and simvastatin has even been employed as a potential therapy for portal hypertension.

So what are the recommendations for liver test monitoring in patients on a statin? The current label for lovastatin no longer requires routine liver test monitoring in the absence of known liver disease. The label suggests monitoring liver tests only if there is a history of liver disease or if there are clinical signs or symptoms of liver disease. For simvastatin and pravastatin, the guidance is similar—just follow liver tests "if clinically indicated." For fluvastatin, atorvastatin, and rosuvastatin, the guidance is to check liver tests before and 12 weeks after the initiation of therapy and "periodically (e.g., semiannually)" thereafter. But there is no reason to stop the drug, especially if the ALT elevations remain below 3 times ULN.

Here's the Point!

If you are asked to stop a statin because of hepatotoxicity concerns, the answer is more often than not "No."

Vignette 23: Big Knuckles

A 39-year-old Caucasian woman presents with complaints of hand discomfort with "big and swollen knuckles." She enjoys fishing and has had more difficulty using her reel. She states that she had an "early menopause" and has been amenorrheic for the past 4 years. She emphasizes that she has a very healthy lifestyle and diet. She loves to eat fresh seafood and takes an assortment of vitamins daily to keep herself "healthy."

On examination, you find that her skin appears tanned, there is no hepatosplenomegaly, and there are no stigmata of chronic liver disease. Her BMI is 32. Hand X-rays reveal degenerative arthritis of her second and third metacarpophalangeal (MCP) and proximal interphalangeal (PIP) joints. Fasting laboratory tests reveal an iron saturation of 75%, ferritin = 432, INR = 1.0, total bilirubin = 0.9, creatinine = 0.8, glucose = 130, albumin = 4.1, ALT = 19, AST = 23, ALP = 98, WBC = 5.8, hemoglobin = 13.9, platelets = 225, with negative autoimmune and viral hepatitis serologies.

▶ **What is the diagnosis?**

▶ **What testing should be performed to confirm the diagnosis?**

▶ **Will treatment help her knuckles?**

▶ **What can you tell the patient about life expectancy?**

▶ **What lifestyle adjustments should you recommend?**

Vignette 23: Answer

This clinical scenario is consistent with hereditary hemochromatosis, an autosomal recessive disorder that leads to excessive intestinal iron absorption due to genetic mutations (most commonly in the *HFE* gene). You probably knew that already, which is good. But the Board exam probably will not ask you simply to diagnose hereditary hemochromatosis; it will probably ask some more nuanced questions, and that is why we are taking this opportunity to review the classic clinical pearls of hemochromatosis.

The clinical manifestations of hemochromatosis arise from excessive iron deposition in the liver, pancreas, heart, and pituitary gland. This woman presented with skin hyperpigmentation, which is present in many patients with hemochromatosis (even at the early stages), prominently on sun-exposed regions of the skin. The skin changes result from iron deposition and increased melanin synthesis in melanocytes. The patient also presents with diabetes, which can be caused by iron accumulation in the pancreatic beta cells in the islets of Langerhans and is present in up to half of hemochromatosis patients. Remember the classic "bronze diabetes" sign of hemochromatosis that you learned in medical school? Both components of "bronze diabetes"—namely, cutaneous hyperpigmentation and hyperglycemia—can improve with phlebotomy. However, phlebotomy does *not* generally help arthropathy, decompensated cirrhosis, or hypogonadism from excess iron deposition in the pituitary. Therefore, this patient's menses are unlikely to resume after phlebotomy, and her arthropathy probably won't improve either. Furthermore, keep in mind that the arthropathy does not correlate with the severity of liver disease.

Serum *HFE* mutation genotype testing is the next step in diagnosing this patient. Since the diagnosis can be readily established in this case with a simple laboratory test (when other options are possible such as liver biopsy), this makes for a great test question. Liver biopsy was previously the gold standard for diagnosis, but it's no longer needed in all patients.

You might be asking, "But how do we know she does not have cirrhosis?" You might feel comfortable diagnosing hemochromatosis without a biopsy, but how can you rule out cirrhosis without performing a biopsy? It turns out that cirrhosis is very rare in hemochromatosis if the AST is normal, there is no hepatomegaly, the ferritin is less than 1000 ng/mL, and the patient is less than 40 years old. Thus, it's unlikely that this patient has cirrhosis, and a liver biopsy and its inherent risks can be avoided.

There are further practical implications as well. For example, this patient may be denied life insurance on the basis of hemochromatosis. However, you can help appeal to the life insurance company that her life expectancy is similar to that of age-matched controls, assuming she is compliant with phlebotomy, if she does not have advanced fibrosis on biopsy. So, after all, you might end up getting a liver biopsy to prognosticate for her life insurance purposes.

Contrary to this case, women tend to present later than men with symptomatic hemochromatosis, since menses provide a route of iron depletion. This patient presented with "early menopause"; however, she was likely amenorrheic due to pituitary iron deposition. A classic Board factlet is that hemochromatosis often remains undetected in women until after menopause. Men tend to develop sequelae far earlier than women do.

Iron in the liver is primarily deposited in periportal hepatocytes in hemochromatosis. As the disease progresses, iron is deposited in the pericentral hepatocytes, macrophages (Kupffer cells), and bile duct cells. In contrast, in a secondary hemosiderosis condition, iron is primarily deposited in macrophages rather than in the hepatocytes. See Vignette 86 for more on the distinction between hemochromatosis and hemosiderosis from secondary iron overload (Figure 23-1).

Of note, there is at least a 20-fold increased risk of hepatocellular carcinoma in patients with hemochromatosis-related cirrhosis (as opposed to the risk in patients with autoimmune hepatitis-related cirrhosis, where hepatocellular carcinoma has only a 1% annual risk). Furthermore, recent data have shown excellent post-transplant survival with hemochromatosis-related cirrhosis (86% at 1 year), similar to that with other causes of cirrhosis. This is in contrast to earlier reports in which the outcomes were not as favorable. However, patients can still develop cardiovascular complications (cardiomyopathy, congestive heart failure, and arrhythmias from cardiac iron deposition) following liver transplantation.

Important lifestyle changes should be recommended for this patient. She should avoid supplemental vitamin C (ascorbic acid) intake, which can increase free iron, leading to oxidative injury and even rapidly fatal cardiomyopathy when ingested in large amounts. She should also avoid uncooked seafood and ensure that her food is properly cleansed, since certain bacteria (*Vibrio vulnificus, Yersinia enterocolitica, Yersinia pseudotuberculosis, Listeria monocytogenes*) can flourish in an iron-rich serum, which can lead to fatal septicemia.

Why Might This Be Tested? Hereditary hemochromatosis can present with a number of signs and symptoms and can be effectively treated if caught early in its course. It also has important lifestyle implications, and Board examiners want to know that you are thinking beyond the algorithmic approach to this condition and also know about key lifestyle advice for the patient. This condition creates a perfect recipe for a variety of potential Board questions. Nearly every sentence of this answer is testable, so know this section well.

Clinical Threshold Alert: A patient under 40 years of age with a ferritin level of less than 1000 ng/mL is unlikely to have cirrhosis, and liver biopsy can often be avoided.

Figure 23-1. T-2 weighted MRI image shows the low signal intensity in the liver compared with the normal spleen signal intensity in hemochromatosis.

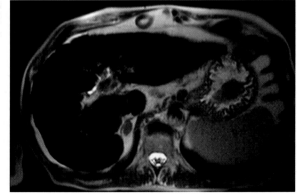

Here's the Point!

"Bronze diabetes" + Arthropathy + High ferritin = Hereditary hemochromatosis

Vignette 24: Abdominal Rash

A 52-year-old man is receiving interferon and ribavirin therapy for chronic hepatitis C infection. Four weeks into his therapeutic course, he presents for follow-up and is found to have a new lesion on his abdomen, pictured in Figure 24-1. No other lesions are noted, and his mucous membranes are unremarkable.

Figure 24-1. Abdominal lesion for Vignette 24.

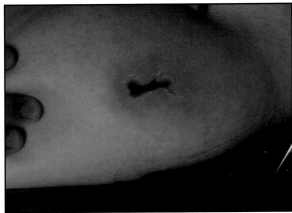

▶ **What is this?**

▶ **What are you going to do about it?**

Vignette 24: Answer

This is a cutaneous reaction to interferon (IFN) injections. You might have known that right off the bat if you've seen it before, but serious injection reactions to IFN are relatively unusual. You might have thought about other HCV-related skin abnormalities, such as porphyria cutanea tarda (PCT) or mixed cryoglobulinemia with a leukocytoclastic vasculitis. However, those reactions look different, as will be described later in this discussion.

Tissue damage at the site of injection is observed with all of the different forms of IFN, although at different rates. The reaction is most common in patients who always use the same injection site; for this reason it's important to instruct patients to rotate their injection site and never use the same site twice in a row. Patients should also avoid injection sites near the waistline, where irritation is more common. The injection site in this photograph is actually just fine—between the navel and waistline.

Injection site reactions occur in up to 60% of patients on IFN, but they are usually not severe. The most common reaction is local erythema. More significant damage involves local tissue damage or necrosis (as pictured), which can be further complicated by localized cellulitis. In this case, the patient did have evidence of surrounding cellulitis and was treated with cephalexin. The IFN was not discontinued—he did fine after rotating his site and being treated for cellulitis.

However, the spectrum of cutaneous adverse effects goes beyond localized necrosis and cellulitis. In fact, the package insert for pegylated IFN alfa-2a states that "serious skin reactions including vesiculobullous eruptions, reactions in the spectrum of Stevens Johnson syndrome (erythema multiforme major) with varying degrees of skin and mucosal involvement and exfoliative dermatitis (erythroderma) have been rarely reported in patients receiving PEG-IFN alfa-2a with and without ribavirin." The insert goes on to say that "patients developing signs or symptoms of severe skin reactions must discontinue therapy." With less severe reactions such as the one pictured, discontinuation is not mandatory. The patient should start by rotating the site of injection, continuing to stay away from the waistline. If site reactions persist despite this maneuver, and especially if there is persistent cellulitis or other complications, then discontinuation is generally warranted, although that decision is usually a case-by-case determination.

While we are in the neighborhood of HCV and skin lesions, we should review a few other important dermatologic associations of HCV and its treatment. For example, ribavirin is also strongly associated with various skin reactions. The dermatological side effects of ribavirin usually occur early in the treatment period and may be due to histamine-like reactions to the agent. Patients describe various types of ribavirin-related rashes spanning from localized erythema to confluent erythematous rashes and vesicular lesions. Some patients also describe itchiness, nasal stuffiness, and even asthma-like symptoms—also probably histamine related. Because the rashes are thought to be histamine mediated, some recommend using topical therapies such as 1% hydrocortisone or triamcinolone. If such interventions do not work, then discontinuation of ribavirin is warranted, which usually leads to clearing of the skin lesions.

As for PCT, this topic could fill a book. But the short story is that PCT is the most common of the various hepatic porphyrias. There are both sporadic and autosomal dominant inherited forms of PCT. In both forms, there is reduced activity of uroporphyrinogen decarboxylase (also known as UROD), which leads to a buildup of uroporphyrinogen in the blood. We could put a figure in this vignette to show you the relevant metabolic pathways, but we're guessing you either already know it (through some miracle of brute memorization or hands-on research in the area), or will never know it. Most people fall in the latter category, so we're just being realistic by keeping that figure out of the book since it's unlikely to show up on the Boards. Our focus here is on the characteristic dermatologic manifestations that can occur when uroporphyrinogen backs up in the blood. Patients with PCT classically have skin reactions that occur in response to sun exposure. The typical PCT lesion consists of vesicles and bullae on the dorsal aspects of the hands. Other sun-exposed areas, such as the face, legs, dorsa of the feet, and forearms, are frequently involved.

Leukocytoclastic vasculitis, another HCV-related skin abnormality, typically presents with palpable purpura in the lower extremities in the setting of underlying mixed cryoglobulinemia. Hepatitis C is the most common cause of cryoglobulinemia. Up to half of patients with hepatitis C have detectable cryoglobulins, although most patients do not suffer consequences from these temperature-sensitive, circulating immunoglobulins. Cryoglobulins precipitate out of solution at temperatures below 98.6°F and can redissolve when rewarmed. This is relevant because cryoglobulins can precipitate out of solution while in blood vessels, leading to a wide range of seemingly disparate consequences, including arthritis, glomerulonephritis, neuropathy, abdominal pain from bowel vasculitis, and a leukocytoclastic vasculitis. Cryoglobulinemia is also marked by low C4 levels and a positive rheumatoid factor. So the presence of any of these features plus some skin lesions in HCV should make you think of cryoglobulinemia.

Why Might This Be Tested? Board examiners seem to love testing on dermatologic manifestations of underlying illness, and they love testing on hepatitis C. So the combination makes for a perfect storm.

Here's the Point!

> Hepatitis C + Interferon treatment + Infraumbilical necrotic lesion/cellulitis = Interferon injection adverse reaction

Here's the Point!

> Hepatitis C + Interferon treatment + Confluent erythematous rashes or vesicles + Pruritus = Ribavirin adverse reaction

Here's the Point!

Hepatitis C + Bullae and vesicles on sun-exposed skin =
Porphyria cutanea tarda

Here's the Point!

Hepatitis C + Lower extremity purpuric rash + Paresthesias + Positive rheumatoid factor + Low complement + Renal disease = Mixed cryoglobulinemia

Vignette 25: Liver Lesion With Central Scar

A 24-year-old woman presents with persistent right upper quadrant (RUQ) discomfort for the past several months and tells you that she "feels something underneath" her ribs. There has been no jaundice, weight loss, or fevers. She has no other significant medical history. Laboratory tests, including liver panel and AFP, are normal. Cross-sectional imaging reveals a noncirrhotic liver with an 8 cm lesion with calcifications within a central scar, as depicted in Figure 25-1.

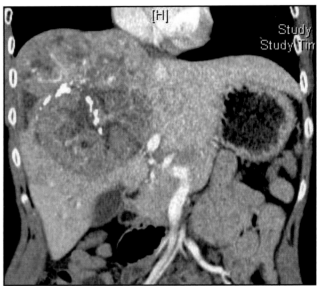

Figure 25-1. Abdominal CT of the patient in Vignette 25. (Reprinted with permission of Barbara Kadell, MD, UCLA Medical Center.)

▶ **What is the diagnosis?**

▶ **What should you recommend?**

Vignette 25: Answer

The best answer is probably not the most obvious: fibrolamellar hepatocellular carcinoma (FLHCC). Your first thought may have been that this is a benign diagnosis of focal nodular hyperplasia (FNH). The "central scar" is the usual Board buzzword for FNH. However, it's extremely rare to have calcifications with FNH, even if there is a central scar. Calcification with a central scar highly suggests the more ominous lesion of FLHCC. Also, on T2-weighted images on MRI, the central scar of FLHCC is dark or hypointense, whereas the central scar of FNH is bright or hyperintense. Steady enlargement of this lesion, if resection were delayed, would also imply the diagnosis of FLHCC.

This patient represents a typical clinical scenario seen with FLHCC (a young patient with vague and persistent RUQ pain, normal synthetic function, and a large lesion found on imaging). It's uncommon (less than 20%) to have an elevated AFP with FLHCC, so the patient's normal AFP value also supports this diagnosis. This lesion is found equally in both young men and women. Treatment consists of aggressive surgical resection, which provides a 5-year survival of around 75%—a value that is surprisingly similar to that for the usual HCC. However, resection is typically more feasible in FLHCC (as opposed to HCC) due to the normal underlying synthetic function of the liver. Figure 25-2 demonstrates a surgical specimen of FLHCC. Look closely: The surrounding liver appears pretty normal; it's not cirrhotic. In contrast, a typical HCC often occurs in the setting of background cirrhosis. Notice that the central scarring is apparent even on the macroscopic appearance of the lesion. Figure 25-3 shows the microscopy of the FLHCC lesion. Compared to HCC, FLHCC has bigger, more granular cells, along with so-called pale bodies and fibrous bands.

FNH is the second most common benign tumor of the liver behind hemangiomas. FNH consists of complexes of benign hepatocytes separated by fibrous bands with prominent bile duct proliferation and malformed blood vessels typically within a central scar. This lesion rarely requires resection unless markedly symptomatic. Since more than half of FNH lesions have a central scar, you can bet that an FNH on the exam will have a central scar. Figure 25-4 depicts an FNH.

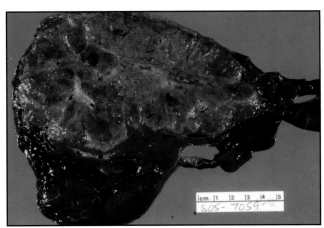

Figure 25-2. Resected fibrolamellar hepatocellular carcinoma (FLHCC). Notice the lack of cirrhosis in the surrounding, normal-appearing parenchyma. Whereas typical HCC occurs in the setting of cirrhosis, FLHCC usually occurs without underlying cirrhosis. There is a central scar with calcification that is consistent with the CT imaging in Figure 25-1. (Reprinted with permission of Charles Lassman, MD, UCLA Medical Center.)

Figure 25-3. Microscopy of FLHCC lesion demonstrating large, granular cells with intervening fibrous bands. (Reprinted with permission of Charles Lassman, MD, UCLA Medical Center.)

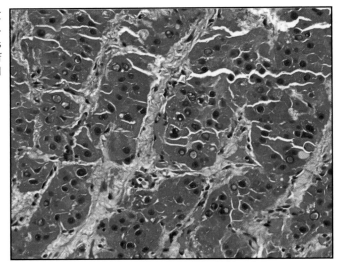

The differential diagnosis could include the following:

- Hemangioma
- Hepatic adenoma
- Hepatocellular carcinoma (usual type)
- Cholangiocarcinoma
- Metastasis

Figure 25-4. Arterial phase from triphasic CT scan of a focal nodular hyperplasia lesion with a characteristic central scar. This is a very different lesion from FLHCC. (Reprinted with permission of Javier Casillas, MD, University of Miami.)

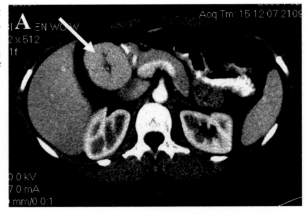

However, the other lesions on this differential typically do not have a central scar and thus would not be good choices to select on a multiple-choice question on a Board exam.

Why Might This Be Tested? This is a case where the imaging provides guidance for therapy. This was cancer and required resection—a very different course of action than what might occur in FNH. Liver lesions are one of the most frequent reasons for consultation with a gastroenterologist. Thus, you need to know this for real life and are very likely to encounter liver lesions on the Board exam.

Here's the Point!

Calcification with a central scar suggests FLHCC rather than FNH.

Vignette 26: Alcohol Binge and a Portal Vein Thrombus

A 26-year-old Latina woman presents to the emergency department with weakness, fatigue, and progressive jaundice over a 2-week period. She reports over 10 years of "heavy" alcohol use since she was a young teenager. She recently went on a drinking binge that culminated in nonbloody vomiting and abdominal swelling (but not pain), in addition to her other chief complaints.

On examination in the emergency room, she is found to be alert to person, place, and time but easily distracted. Her vital signs reveal a temperature of 99.9°F, blood pressure of 128/72, heart rate of 112, and respiratory rate of 18 with 98% oxygen saturation on room air. She has scleral icterus, mild conjunctival pallor, and sublingual icterus. There is no cervical lymphadenopathy. Her lungs are clear, and her heart is tachycardic but without murmurs. Her abdomen reveals moderate distention but no fluid wave or shifting dullness on percussion. Her abdomen is otherwise soft and nontender. Rectal exam yields brown stool. There is 1+ lower extremity pitting edema. There are no spider angiomas and no palmar erythema. Neurologic examination is nonfocal; there is no asterixis. Laboratories include the following: WBC = 33.4 with 92% PMNs, INR = 1.8, prothrombin time = 15.4, creatinine = 2.1, albumin = 2.8, total bilirubin = 19.8, AST = 151, ALT = 74, ALP = 164. Ultrasound performed in the emergency department reveals a large fatty liver, enlarged spleen, and evidence of hepatofugal flow with a portal vein thrombus. There are no stones in the gallbladder, and the common bile duct is 4 mm in diameter. She is now admitted to your service from the emergency department for further inpatient management.

▶ **What is the most likely diagnosis?**

▶ **What will your treatment plan be?**

▶ **How are you going to handle the portal vein thrombus?**

Vignette 26: Answer

This is acute alcoholic hepatitis (AH) in the setting of underlying chronic liver disease. Although this patient is young, she still can have chronic liver disease or even outright cirrhosis. When this patient arrived in the emergency department, there was confusion about what was going on. Was this just acute AH? Or was there underlying cirrhosis as well? Wasn't she too young to have cirrhosis? And what about this portal vein thrombus? Did the thrombus need to be actively treated? Was there something else altogether underlying this pattern of liver injury, like autoimmune hepatitis, acute viral hepatitis, and so forth? (The patient had no records on file at the time of her emergency room visit.) Or was this just an impacted gallstone?

Before we get to those questions, it's important to review the spectrum of alcohol-related liver damage. The usual range of liver injury begins with simple steatosis, which could evolve to steatohepatitis, which could ultimately lead to early fibrosis and outright cirrhosis. But these stages are not mutually exclusive or distinct. The spectrum of liver injury does not follow a perfectly linear path, but instead can be erratic and overlapping. Some people exhibit different forms of liver injury at once. In this patient, who unfortunately died after a prolonged inpatient hospitalization, the autopsy revealed evidence of alcoholic liver disease (ie, Mallory bodies, megamitochondria, inflammatory infiltrate) and early perisinusoidal fibrosis, but not cirrhosis (ie, no evidence of regenerative nodules with bridging fibrosis). Yet when she presented to the emergency room, there was evidence of portal hypertension, as indicated by the ascites, hepatofugal flow on ultrasound, and a portal vein thrombus (more on that later). Alcohol is known to transiently increase portal pressures, so even if a patient does not harbor outright cirrhosis, she can appear to have cirrhosis in the setting of acute alcohol toxicity. The woman in this vignette had portal hypertension, fibrosis (but not outright cirrhosis), and evidence of acute AH, supported by the high AST:ALT ratio (well over the traditional 2:1 ratio seen in acute AH), leukocytosis, and high Maddrey discriminant function (DF) score driven by the elevated INR and total bilirubin (more on the DF score later).

Fatty liver is common in people who drink a lot of alcohol. This can show up on ultrasonography when there is more than 30% steatosis in the liver. In fact, up to 90% of people who consume more than 60 g of alcohol per day have steatosis. In the United States, the standard "drink," which includes a 12-oz can of beer, 5-oz glass of wine, or 1.5-oz shot of hard liquor, contains roughly 12 g of alcohol by weight. (By the way, Japan tends to have the "strongest" drinks by average alcohol content.) So 60 g of daily alcohol ingestion equates to around 5 drinks per day. Almost everyone who drinks this much alcohol has hepatic steatosis.

The progression to advanced liver injury depends on several variables. Gender is an especially strong predictor of alcohol-induced liver injury; women are generally more susceptible to the hepatotoxic effects of alcohol than men due to gender-related enzymatic differences. Whereas it often takes 60 g of alcohol per day for around 10 years for men to progress to chronic injury, it may take only 20 g per day to achieve the same effect for women. This may well explain how this patient, who was only 26 years old, had already developed advanced fibrosis. Another factor that predicts liver injury is the pattern in which alcohol is ingested. Data indicate that binge drinkers (like this woman) have a higher incidence of advanced injury and mortality compared to people who drink only during meals, even if the same amount of alcohol is ingested over the long run. So there may be something about getting the hit all at once that really kick-starts the injury cascade. Race may also play a role in predicting liver injury from alcohol. Data reveal that rates of cirrhosis are higher in African-Americans and Latinos than in Caucasians, and alcohol-related mortality is highest in the Latino population, independent of the amount of alcohol consumed. This may reflect racial variations in alcohol dehydrogenase, among other factors both known and unknown. This patient happened to be a Latina woman, so she carried two independent risk factors for accelerated liver injury from alcohol.

Simple steatosis is often fully reversible and usually (but not always) subsides after 6 weeks of abstinence. Unfortunately, even with abstinence some people (up to 15% in some series) still progress to fibrosis and cirrhosis. Once steatosis has set in, it does not take that much more drinking to keep the damage coming. Only 40 g per day of continued drinking (around 3 drinks per day) is enough to progress to fibrosis and cirrhosis in approximately one third of individuals with alcoholic steatosis.

Acute AH itself can range from mild injury to catastrophic, life-threatening illness, as occurred here. It's important to remember that acute steatohepatitis often occurs in the setting of underlying chronic liver disease. The mere presence of acute AH suggests a strong history of drinking and is a surrogate marker for underlying chronic liver injury, not just acute injury. Of note, in the setting of cirrhosis, the traditional AST:ALT ratio of 2:1 does not always hold, so you should still keep AH in mind even if the ratio is different. It's useful to calculate the Maddrey DF score when you suspect AH. The DF is a disease severity score developed years ago to predict mortality. The Board exam will probably not ask you to calculate a DF, and most people have a calculator for this on their handheld devices. But with that said, here is the equation: DF = 4.6 * (Patient's Prothrombin Time − Control Prothrombin Time) + Total Bilirubin. The main thing to remember is that the prothrombin time and total bilirubin are the 2 biochemical factors that predict mortality in AH, at least by the Maddrey DF standard. The risk of mortality shoots up when the score exceeds 32. The MELD score, which is generally used for allocating liver transplants (see Vignette 9), can also be useful to predict outcomes in acute AH; the prognosis is worst when the MELD exceeds 18. Both the DF and MELD scores include prothrombin time (or INR) and total bilirubin levels, although the MELD also includes creatinine. Aminotransaminases are not part of any validated prognostic scores in hepatology, namely because they are not liver function tests, despite commonly being referred to as LFTs. See Vignette 1 for more on that.

If a patient's DF exceeds 32 or MELD exceeds 18 (as in this case), it's time to begin timely medical interventions. Whereas supportive therapy is important for everyone with acute AH (ie, nutritional support with vitamins, monitoring for alcohol withdrawal), more aggressive therapy is needed for patients with a poor prognosis. The usual decision is whether to begin a systemic steroid, such as prednisolone, or anti-TNF therapy, such as pentoxifylline. Both are acceptable, and it would be hard to imagine the Board exam allowing one as a correct answer but not the other. That said, there are a few nuances to know about these different approaches. Regarding steroids, the effect on mortality is small and somewhat controversial (different results in different studies), but the overall effect from meta-analysis is positive, with a number needed to treat of 5 (ie, for every 5 people with AH that you treat with steroids instead of placebo, there is 1 additional survivor) for a short-term mortality benefit. This benefit appears highest in patients with concurrent spontaneous hepatic encephalopathy. Most of the data have been with prednisolone (40 mg per day for 4 weeks followed by a taper), not prednisone. Since the liver is responsible for the conversion of prednisone to the active metabolite prednisolone, which may be challenging in a patient with poor synthetic function, prednisolone has been used more often. A final point is that steroids are associated with more infections than placebo, which undermines their benefit.

As for pentoxifylline, this oral phosphodiesterase inhibitor with anti-TNF activity is associated with a significantly lower risk of mortality than placebo, and is especially effective in the setting of hepatorenal syndrome (HRS). Thus some physicians prefer this therapy when the creatinine is elevated and there is suspicion for underlying HRS (see Vignette 75 for more on HRS). It remains uncertain whether combining both steroids and pentoxifylline is any better than either therapy alone.

What about the portal vein thrombosis? In general, the answer is *usually nothing*. Portal vein thrombosis is typically an epiphenomenon of high intrahepatic pressures in cirrhosis and hepatic fibrosis and is a surrogate marker for hepatofugal (away from the liver) flow. When the intrahepatic pressure rises, the pressure within the portal vein begins to rise in lockstep. After a while, the blood can't flow into the liver (see Figure 3-2), and it starts to back up, become static, and then clot. But the clot, in and of itself, is not necessarily something to target with therapy in this setting. It's one thing if a clot organizes and extends down the mesenteric system. It's also a different situation if there is an underlying prothrombotic condition giving rise to the clot (eg, factor V Leiden). But if the clot is limited to the portal vein, it does not need treatment. In this case, the admitting team began heparin, and after a traumatic paracentesis that lanced a recanalizing umbilical vessel, the patient exsanguinated and required emergency surgery to find the bleeding source and achieve hemostasis. Suffice it to say anticoagulation was not the answer for this particular portal vein thrombus. The answer is abstinence from alcohol (obviously), medical therapy for acute AH, nutritional support, watching for alcohol withdrawal, imaging to ensure that there isn't a complicating HCC with portal vein invasion, and monitoring (and hoping) for biochemical evidence of improvement. Heparin did not have a role in this setting. The admitting diagnosis from the emergency department was not alcoholic hepatitis; it was portal vein thrombus. By mistaking an epiphenomenon as the reason for admission, the entire focus of the admission was on the clot itself. The patient did not receive steroids or pentoxifylline. She was very ill, so it remains unclear if the therapy would have helped, but the point is to make the diagnosis quickly, begin appropriate therapy right away in the setting of an elevated DF or MELD score, and provide supportive therapy throughout.

Why Might This Be Tested? Everyone manages patients with acute AH, but not everyone is good at diagnosing it. For such a common problem, it's surprising how frequently acute AH is misdiagnosed and mismanaged. In this case, for example, the patient had a low-grade fever and persistent leukocytosis with a left shift that triggered an extensive workup. The workup not only included blood cultures and other expeditions for underlying infection, but even included a bone marrow biopsy to screen for myeloproliferative disorders! In fact, this patient was also treated empirically with broad-spectrum antibiotics. Yet leukocytosis and low-grade fevers are classic features of acute AH; they are part of the illness itself.

Another common situation is for a patient with AH to have an elevated ALP along with the high total bilirubin, as occurred here. This almost inevitably leads to an ultrasound and request for an endoscopic retrograde cholangiopancreatography (ERCP) to screen for an impacted stone. Although acute AH frequently presents with a high ALP and total bilirubin, the presentation is otherwise totally different from that with an impacted stone, where there would typically be a higher ALT than AST (see Vignette 32), and where there would be a characteristic pattern of biliary colic. The bottom line is that it should not be hard to distinguish acute AH from an impacted gallstone. If this vignette were on a Board exam and you were asked for the diagnosis, the answer would be acute AH, as it would usually be in real life also. So just make the AH diagnosis and get started with appropriate therapy (while, of course, keeping a broad differential diagnosis in the back of your mind).

Clinical Threshold Alerts: If the AST:ALT ratio exceeds 2:1 in the setting of recent alcohol ingestion, think about acute AH. A "standard drink" in the United States contains roughly 12 to 14 g of alcohol by weight. Ingesting 60 g of alcohol per day for 10 years can lead to cirrhosis in men, whereas ingesting only 20 g per day can lead to cirrhosis in many women. If the Maddrey DF score exceeds 32, or if the MELD exceeds 18, then initiate either prednisolone or pentoxifylline in acute AH. If there is more than 30% hepatic steatosis, it can be detected by ultrasonography.

Here's the Point!

↑ WBC + ↑ Total bilirubin + ↑ ALP + Low-grade fever + ↑ Alcohol = Think about acute alcoholic hepatitis, not just a gallstone or cholangitis!

Here's the Point!

Portal vein thrombus in cirrhosis or acute alcoholic hepatitis? Treat the underlying disease, not the epiphenomenon.

Vignette 27: Empty Pill Bottle

A 23-year-old woman is brought into the emergency department by paramedics after she was found lying on the floor next to an empty acetaminophen bottle in her apartment. Her father had not heard from her after speaking to her 2 nights ago when she was upset after a recent breakup with her boyfriend. She is noted to be jaundiced and lethargic with unremarkable vital signs. Laboratory tests reveal the following: pH = 7.23, INR = 3.1, total bilirubin = 16.1, creatinine = 2.8, AST = 7210, ALT = 6590, albumin = 3.2, glucose = 52; acetaminophen level is at the minimally detectable range.

▸ *What should you do?*

Vignette 27: Answer

This patient is in serious trouble. She has acute liver failure (ALF) and is at high risk of death given her pH of less than 7.3 (she meets King's College Criteria, as shown in Table 27-1). Although many patients with acetaminophen-induced ALF recover with supportive care, this patient is unlikely to survive without orthotopic liver transplantation. You need to take action quickly, and the patient needs to be referred to a liver transplant center immediately. Transportation can be dangerous, in and of itself, if there is increased intracranial pressure and/or severe coagulopathy. Also, the liver transplant center will need time to perform an expedited transplant evaluation. So when the patient is in bad shape, you (and the patient) need to move quickly!

Okay, so the patient is getting admitted to the ICU and has been referred to a transplant center. But, she will need treatment. Remember that acetaminophen is a dose-dependent toxin that can cause ALF typically when more than 7.5 to 8 g are ingested. However, the hepatotoxicity is enhanced in patients who are concomitantly taking isoniazid, rifampin, phenytoin, or carbamazepine, and in alcoholics, due to induction of the cytochrome P450 system. Furthermore, there will be more damage in a fasting or malnourished state due to glutathione depletion.

Table 27-1.
KING'S COLLEGE HOSPITAL CRITERIA FOR LIVER TRANSPLANTATION
Acetaminophen-Induced Acute Liver Failure
Arterial pH <7.3 (irrespective of the grade of encephalopathy)   OR   Creatinine >3.4 and INR >6.5 and grade 3 or 4 encephalopathy
Non-Acetaminophen-Induced Acute Liver Failure
INR >6.5 (irrespective of the grade of encephalopathy)   OR   Any 3 of the following: 1. Age <10 years or >40 years   2. Etiology: Idiosyncratic drug reactions, halothane hepatitis, non-A hepatitis, non-B hepatitis   3. Duration of jaundice before encephalopathy >1 week   4. INR >3.5   5. Bilirubin >18 mg/dL
* You don't need to memorize this table (that would be fair game for the transplant hepatology examination, not the GI exam). However, you should know the basics.

Therefore, lesser amounts can also cause ALF in some patients. In the United States there are also analgesic medications that combine acetaminophen (a dose-dependent hepatotoxin) with an addictive narcotic in a single tablet (eg, Vicodin, Percocet). Doesn't really make sense to bundle them, does it? Taking too many of these tablets (due to excessive pain or addiction) can accidentally lead to ALF—the so-called therapeutic misadventure. Even though 48 hours may have transpired since this patient ingested the acetaminophen, there may still be a benefit to using N-acetylcysteine (NAC) therapy. Depending upon the clinical scenario, NAC can be administered either orally or intravenously per standard protocol. Risk of injury can be estimated with the acetaminophen nomogram, shown in Figure 27-1, but this is not something that needs to be memorized for the GI Board exam. You can also throw the nomogram out the window if you have an alcoholic patient or if they are on medications that can induce the cytochrome p450 system. That's really important to remember: The nomogram is uninterpretable in an alcoholic with acetaminophen toxicity.

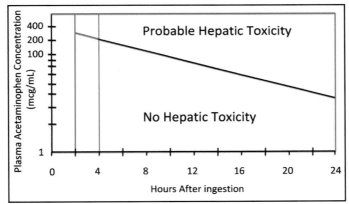

Figure 27-1. Acetaminophen toxicity nomogram. (Reprinted with permission of Dheeresh J. Patel, MA.)

Ipecac is not indicated in this patient due to risk of aspiration with emesis, since she is obtunded, and also because this was not a recent ingestion. But, if the time of ingestion would have been in the past few hours, then activated charcoal would have been indicated. However, if charcoal is administered, then it must be given well before oral NAC to avoid problems with absorption.

ALF is defined as acute severe liver injury of less than 6 months' duration with impaired synthetic function, coagulopathy, and encephalopathy in a patient with a previously normal liver or well-compensated liver disease (such as Wilson disease, hepatitis B, or autoimmune hepatitis). Previously used terms such as *fulminant hepatic failure* and *hyperacute or subacute liver failure* are not typically used any longer since they do not help predict prognosis. The etiology is much more important than the length of illness. For example, "hyperacute" liver failure from acetaminophen generally has a better prognosis than "subacute" liver failure from an idiosyncratic drug reaction.

Acetaminophen is the most common cause of ALF in the United States and Europe (where it's called paracetamol). You should also know that certain etiologies tend to do better than others; liver failure from acetaminophen, hepatitis A, and hepatitis B all have a better prognosis than liver failure from Wilson disease, autoimmune hepatitis, idiosyncratic drug-induced liver injury, or indeterminate etiology.

Why Might This Be Tested? Acute liver failure is one of the classic emergencies for which the gastroenterologist can be awakened in the middle of the night by a call from the emergency department. Acetaminophen is the most common cause of ALF, so you are bound to see this on an exam and in real life.

Clinical Threshold Alert: A pH of <7.3 in acetaminophen-induced ALF is an indication for liver transplantation listing. And be aware of the various King's College Criteria (more on this later in this book as well).

Here's the Point!

Very high INR + Severe hepatic encephalopathy → Severe synthetic dysfunction → Dismal prognosis without liver transplantation

Vignette 28: Elevated Aminotransaminases on a Routine Physical Exam

A 41-year-old Caucasian woman is referred for evaluation of persistently elevated liver tests. She was initially found to have an ALT of 92 and an AST of 83 on routine tests as part of a physical examination. Her liver function tests, including INR, total bilirubin, and albumin, have all been normal. She underwent evaluation for various forms of hepatitis, which has been negative to date. Specifically, there is no biochemical evidence of infection with hepatitis A, B, or C, and her ANA is negative. A right upper quadrant ultrasound was normal.

The patient's past medical history is remarkable for iron-deficiency anemia thought to be from menorrhagia as well as irritable bowel syndrome (IBS). She has not received a colonoscopy or upper endoscopy. She takes intermittent ibuprofen for aches and pains. She does not use any herbal therapies or alternative medicinal preparations.

A review of systems reveals intermittent painful oral ulcers, recurrent lower abdominal cramping that improves with bowel movements, intermittent diarrhea, and chronic fatigue. She has no children, although she tried for years to conceive and had an infertility workup that did not identify an underlying cause.

Physical exam reveals a thin patient with a BMI of 18. There is no icterus or stigmata of chronic liver disease. There are scattered aphthous ulcerations along the bilateral buccal mucosa. There is no lymphadenopathy. Abdominal exam does not reveal hepatosplenomegaly, masses, or tenderness. Rectal examination reveals brown loose stool that is heme-negative. The remainder of her examination is unremarkable.

▶ *What diagnostic test should you order next?*

Vignette 28: Answer

This patient needs to be screened for celiac sprue, either with an anti-tissue transglutaminase IgA or anti-endomysial IgA antibody. Celiac sprue is one of those conditions that seems to do just about everything; you can put it on virtually any morning report differential diagnosis and be right. It should be tested here because of its association with elevations in aminotransferase levels. The exact mechanism for this association remains unclear, but it's well known that more than 40% of patients with celiac sprue have abnormally elevated aminotransferase levels. In contrast, celiac patients do not typically have abnormal liver *function* tests, such as total bilirubin, INR, or albumin (unless there is a concurrent liver process accompanying the sprue). Furthermore, up to 10% of patients with unexplained elevations in AST and ALT have underlying celiac sprue. All of this supports testing for sprue in this patient. The elevated liver tests usually normalize after starting a gluten-free diet.

In this case there are many reasons to suspect underlying celiac sprue, in addition to the lab values. The patient is Caucasian, which is the first tip-off. In addition, she has long-standing iron-deficiency anemia, recurrent aphthous oral ulcerations, a diagnosis of IBS (celiac disease occurs in around 1% to 4% of IBS patients), and infertility. Plus her physical exam reveals a thin body habitus, which suggests possible nutrient malabsorption. An abdominal ultrasound may be consistent with fatty liver and will also show hyposplenism (small spleen) in celiac disease, supported by the presence of Howell-Jolly bodies on the peripheral smear. Given all of this, it would be a major mistake to forget about testing for sprue. Making the diagnosis of sprue could have large positive impact on the patient's overall quality of life, not just her liver test abnormalities.

Why Might This Be Tested? It's estimated that around 1 in every 133 Americans has celiac sprue. Whether or not that precise number is true, it's clear that sprue is a prevalent condition that is frequently missed. Board examiners will want to know that you can make this diagnosis on a timely basis. But it would be too easy to just show a Marsh 3 lesion in this patient and ask for the diagnosis; instead, the examiners will likely want to see if you can recognize less common (although still common) presentations of celiac sprue—in this case, elevated aminotransferase levels. Finally, Board examiners have a number of content "check boxes" they need to check off when putting an exam together. This topic works well because it covers several areas, including both luminal GI and liver disease. With one question they could potentially test across several content areas.

Here's the Point!

> **Unexplained elevated aminotransferases + Any of the following:**
> - Iron-deficiency anemia
> - Infertility
> - Osteoporosis
> - Itchy elbow rashes (dermatitis herpetiformis)
> - IBS symptoms
> - Etc, etc, etc...
>
> **Think celiac sprue!**

Vignette 29: Still Yellow

You are asked to evaluate a 39-year-old man who developed hepatitis A virus (HAV) infection 3 months ago. At the time, he had returned from a month-long beach vacation, during which he ate raw seafood. He initially presented with low-grade fever, malaise, diarrhea, anorexia, right upper quadrant discomfort, and jaundice. His blood tests at the time of acute infection included the following: total bilirubin = 6.8, ALT = 1987, and AST = 1492. He felt better soon thereafter but noticed that his skin was yellow despite otherwise feeling markedly better. He saw his primary care provider in follow-up yesterday, who advised him to see you urgently. The patient mentions that his doctor "was freaking out since I was still yellow and he wanted me to see you again to do more tests right away." Laboratory tests from yesterday are notable for a total bilirubin = 8.9, ALT = 1987, and AST = 70.

▶ **What is going on here?**

▶ **What test(s) should you order?**

Vignette 29: Answer

This is prolonged cholestasis (aka cholestatic hepatitis) from HAV infection and is one of the often forgotten, atypical manifestations of HAV (notice the term *acute* is not needed before HAV since there is no "chronic" HAV infection). In typical HAV infection, patients may develop a prodrome of anorexia, malaise, fever, nausea, diarrhea, and right upper quadrant pain. Days later they can have pruritus and icterus, and diagnosis is confirmed with serum HAV IgM. Of note, jaundice occurs in about 30% of adults but is much less common in children with HAV. The rise in bilirubin occurs after the initial marked elevation of the ALT and AST. Typically, the bilirubin gradually falls to normal within 3 months. However, some patients may develop this prolonged cholestasis variant of HAV infection, where the bilirubin can be markedly elevated (more than 10 mg/dL) before finally returning to normal spontaneously over the next 3 to 5 months. Patience is the key here, since the deep jaundice will resolve on its own without long-term sequelae. A short course of steroids (prednisolone) could be an option to shorten the cholestatic picture if the patient were having marked pruritus, weight loss, or anorexia. However, there have been reports of steroid use precipitating HAV relapse (more on relapse in a moment). Regardless, steroids are not indicated for this patient since he is asymptomatic; expectant care is best. Remember that old clinical saying, "Jaundice [by itself] never kills anyone," or the common variant, "Jaundice [by itself] is merely cosmetic."

Regarding further testing, an HAV IgM can be ordered (which often would still be positive) if you are unsure of the original diagnosis, but is not absolutely necessary to make the diagnosis. You might also consider a right upper quadrant ultrasound to exclude biliary obstruction. Beyond this, nothing else should be needed diagnostically. It's reasonable in this case to recommend to the primary care physician that you would just sit tight, let nature take its course, and expect a complete recovery. In fact, invasive testing, such as liver biopsy or ERCP, could cause unnecessary complications and expense.

Relapsing hepatitis is another atypical clinical manifestation of HAV infection with a self-explanatory name. After HAV seemingly resolves with normalization of liver tests and symptoms, there can be a "relapse" a few weeks later with symptoms and laboratory tests similar to those in the initial phase, including HAV IgM in the serum and even HAV isolated in the stool. The general rule is that this also resolves spontaneously. HAV is one of the success stories in public health. Due to improvements in public health measures such as sanitation and immunization, the incidence of HAV has been decreasing steadily in the United States.

Why Might This Be Tested? HAV is a classic illness, but atypical manifestations of the disease are often forgotten and lead to unnecessary tests that have their own inherent risks and expenses. Therefore it's prudent to recognize this atypical presentation of HAV.

Here's the Point!

> Prolonged cholestasis and relapsing hepatitis are atypical manifestations of HAV and resolve spontaneously.

Vignette 30: Trouble During a Steroid Taper

A 52-year-old man presented to his primary care physician with painful erythematous nodules on his anterior shins and recurrent abdominal pain. After evaluation, he was found to have polyarteritis nodosa (PAN) complicated by abdominal and renal vasculitis. He was started on high-dose prednisone, which led to symptomatic improvement. After steroid induction was complete, the patient began a slow taper off steroids. Four weeks later, he noticed that his eyes were yellow, which was quickly followed by yellow skin and overwhelming fatigue. He presented to the emergency department, where he was found to be deeply jaundiced with tender hepatomegaly on examination. Laboratory values included the following: AST = 1208, ALT = 1633, LDH = 521, total bilirubin = 22.3, INR = 3.8, creatinine = 1.6, albumin = 3.4. He was admitted to the hospital, where his condition rapidly deteriorated with the development of advanced encephalopathy, eventually culminating in coma and death.

▶ **What happened here?**

▶ **What diagnostic test should have been done prior to starting steroids?**

Vignette 30: Answer

This is acute liver failure resulting from acute HBV infection in the setting of immune reconstitution. How would you know that this is probably HBV when that was not mentioned in the vignette? You may recall that polyarteritis nodosa (PAN) is frequently associated with HBV and in some cases may be a secondary reaction to chronic infection with HBV. That's an important relationship to remember. Hepatitis C infection has also been associated with PAN, but hepatitis C does not typically lead to acute liver failure in the setting of immune reconstitution. In contrast, dormant HBV is known to spring to life, so to speak, in the setting of immune reconstitution following a period of immune suppression. This has been described in a variety of conditions, including PAN, during withdrawal of steroids. During immune suppression, there is enhancement of HBV replication with diffuse involvement of the hepatocytes. The HBV is primed and ready to attack. As the immune system reconstitutes following steroid withdrawal (or, say, completion of chemotherapy in a different setting), there is a resurgence of cell-mediated immunity that leads to direct injury of the hepatocytes harboring the HBV. This is a natural response to try to rid the body of the rampant HBV, but is quite literally a major overkill. It's like taking a bazooka to an anthill. So the HBV itself does not directly damage the hepatocytes; instead, the cell-mediated immunity itself damages the liver. This injury can range from transient hepatocellular damage to acute liver failure, as seen here. The typical time course is within 2 to 6 weeks following withdrawal of the immune-suppressing agent (eg, steroids, chemotherapy, or anti-TNF therapy). Because HBV is so closely linked to PAN, it's vital to screen for latent HBV prior to beginning steroids, because the withdrawal phase can lead to serious problems if the HBV has not been properly handled.

Why Might This Be Tested? A vignette like this could test several different facts at once, which makes for a good potential Board question. Not only do you need to remember the relationship between PAN and HBV, but you also need to recognize that immune suppression in untreated HBV can lead to severe liver injury and even acute liver failure. Finally, remember that the damage from HBV is not directly caused by the virus, but is indirectly caused by the virus hijacking the innate immunity to wreak havoc on the hepatocytes. For Board exams and life in general, remember that it's important to check for latent HBV prior to immune suppression.

Here's the Point!

Polyarteritis nodosa on a GI Board exam? Think hepatitis B.

Here's the Point!

Acute liver failure upon withdrawal of immune suppression = Think immune-mediated damage orchestrated by HBV

Vignette 31: Abnormal Liver Tests

You are asked to see a 31-year-old woman for abnormal liver tests. She has had malaise and generalized weakness progressively worsening over the past 4 months without fever. She is now so fatigued that she has trouble getting out of her chair. She does not have a history of liver disease, viral hepatitis, jaundice, illicit drug use, prescription drug use, herbal drug use, over-the-counter drug use (including acetaminophen products), alcohol use, or previous abnormal liver tests. She has had liver tests performed annually at her routine health care maintenance visits with her primary care provider, and they have always been normal. Her laboratory tests now reveal elevations in her AST and ALT confirmed on 2 samples. Therefore, you have been asked to provide consultation and perform a liver biopsy.

When you see the patient, physical examination shows no stigmata of chronic liver disease and no rashes. Labs reveal the following: AST = 980, ALT = 490, total bilirubin = 1.0, albumin = 3.4, ALP = 108, WBC = 11.1, hemoglobin = 13.2, platelets = 394, ESR = 42.

Last week the patient had the following tests with normal results: ANA, smooth muscle antibody, anti-liver/kidney microsomal antibody, soluble liver antigen, ceruloplasmin, hepatitis A IgM, hepatitis B core IgM, hepatitis C RNA, hepatitis E IgM, HSV IgM, EBV IgM, CMV IgM, and abdominal ultrasonography.

▶ *What is the diagnosis?*
▶ *What test should you order first?*

Vignette 31: Answer

A simple blood test with serum creatinine kinase (CK) would help to yield the diagnosis, which is polymyositis. In this case, the patient had been seeing her internist for 2 months before we made the diagnosis upon seeing her on the inpatient service. When we tested the patient's CK, it was over 3000. The CK test avoided the need for a liver biopsy. A muscle biopsy confirmed the diagnosis of polymyositis, and the patient dramatically responded to steroid therapy.

Muscle injury of any cause, including rhabdomyolysis, can give a false-positive indication of "acute hepatitis." Muscle contains both AST and ALT, and with injury these can be elevated, with AST typically elevated more than ALT. It's important to think about the patient in a broad sense (including the history) when you are evaluating abnormal liver tests. You are the expert consultant, so you can't have tunnel vision. A liver biopsy is reasonable if the diagnosis is in doubt and can certainly diagnose autoimmune hepatitis. However, a simple blood test (CK) in this case helped to establish the diagnosis and spare the potential risks of a liver biopsy.

Why Might This Be Tested? Since the ABIM creates the examination, anything under the umbrella of internal medicine is fair game for a test question. "Abnormal LFTs" is one of the most common reasons to consult a gastroenterologist. You should know all the potential etiologies of elevated AST and ALT, including nonhepatic etiologies.

Here's the Point!

Elevated AST and ALT can be due to muscle injury and
not necessarily to hepatitis.

Vignette 32: Pancreatitis and Elevated Alanine Aminotransferase

A 38-year-old woman presents to the emergency room with a chief complaint of abdominal pain, nausea, and vomiting. The following labs are noted: amylase = 836, lipase = 562, AST = 132, ALT = 214, ALP = 86, total bilirubin = 1.2.

▶ *Without knowing anything else, what is the most likely cause of the pancreatitis?*

Vignette 32: Answer

This is most likely acute gallstone pancreatitis. The usual debate in acute pancreatitis concerns how best to distinguish between its two most common etiologies: gallstones versus alcohol. Obviously, a history of recent alcohol ingestion is a key fact to support alcohol over gallstones (as compared to the many other etiologies of pancreatitis), but patients' stories are often suboptimal or less than clear-cut. Here you don't have a history to review, so the vignette is really testing your ability to predict gallstone versus alcoholic pancreatitis using biochemical parameters alone (an admittedly artificial exercise, but useful nonetheless).

There are 2 laboratory parameters that are helpful. The first is the serum ALT level. Data indicate that when the ALT exceeds 150 IU/L (roughly 3 to 5 times the upper limit of normal) with elevated pancreatic enzyme levels, the positive predictive value for gallstone pancreatitis is 95%. Said another way, when the ALT is over ~150 in the setting of acute pancreatitis, there is a 95% chance of underlying gallstone pancreatitis, regardless of anything else. In contrast, neither the ALP nor the total bilirubin level is predictive of gallstone pancreatitis. A common misconception is that the ALP and total bilirubin rise before the ALT in the setting of a stone obstructing the common bile duct and/or pancreatic duct. Yet it's the ALT—not the ALP or total bilirubin—that jumps up first. The AST can also be elevated, although its sensitivity and specificity for acute gallstone pancreatitis lag slightly behind those for ALT. The ALP rise can be slow in all forms of acute biliary obstruction because the elevation is from induction and new synthesis of ALP rather than spillage of stored enzymes. So the rise in ALP can take a little time after acute biliary obstruction, whereas aminotransferases tend to rise much faster. Also keep in mind that patients can have gallstone pancreatitis even if an abdominal ultrasound is unrevealing; in acute pancreatitis, there can be overlying bowel gas from ileus that obscures the view. A normal ultrasound should not stop the hunt for a stone, especially when the ALT is elevated.

The second laboratory parameter is the ratio of lipase to amylase. Elevated lipase to amylase ratios, especially when greater than 2.0, are predictive of alcoholic rather than gallstone pancreatitis. The sensitivity and specificity of this rule for predicting alcoholic pancreatitis are 91% and 76%, respectively. For the patient described in this vignette, the ratio is less than 1.0, arguing against alcoholic pancreatitis. But this rule is not carved in stone—it's more of a clinical pearl that is supported by some data but is not widely proven. So it's best to focus mainly on the high ALT. When the ALT is 150 or above in pancreatitis, think gallstones—don't be dissuaded by a normal ALP or total bilirubin.

Why Might This Be Tested? A vignette like this one provides a good way to see if you know a time-tested clinical threshold. Plus it tests whether you have fallen prey to the misconception that a near-normal ALP and/or total bilirubin are incompatible with ductal obstruction. They are not... at all. Board examiners are almost certain to test your general knowledge in interpreting liver tests, and this is a good way to test your knowledge of a sometimes underappreciated use of the ALT, in particular.

Clinical Threshold Alert: If a patient with pancreatitis has an ALT exceeding 150, then he or she probably has gallstone pancreatitis (positive predictive value of 95% based on meta-analysis of multiple studies). In contrast, if the lipase-to-amylase ratio exceeds 2.0, then alcoholic pancreatitis is likely, not gallstone pancreatitis.

Here's the Point!

Pancreatitis + Elevated ALT = Think gallstone pancreatitis

Vignette 33: Primary Biliary Cirrhosis

A 38-year-old woman with primary biliary cirrhosis (PBC) presents for a follow-up examination in the office after the diagnosis was made 6 months ago. She had a percutaneous liver biopsy showing stage 2 fibrosis with a positive antimitochondrial antibody; this was initially performed to evaluate an asymptomatic elevation in her ALP level. She was placed on ursodeoxycholic acid therapy and has remained on a 1000 mg total daily dose. She has been doing well without fatigue, pruritus, abdominal distention, weight loss, confusion, or bleeding, and currently has no complaints. She weighs 70 kg and physical examination is unremarkable. Laboratory tests from earlier today reveal the following: Na = 140, creatinine = 0.8, AST = 17, ALT = 19, total bilirubin = 1.0, ALP = 90, GGT = 35, INR = 1.0, albumin = 4.0, WBC = 6.9, hemoglobin = 13.2, platelets = 124.

▶ **What tests should you recommend?**

Vignette 33: Answer

This patient should have an upper endoscopy despite the lack of cirrhosis on biopsy. Patients with PBC, unlike most other liver diseases, are at risk to develop presinusoidal portal hypertension due to nodular regenerative hyperplasia, even without cirrhosis. Portal hypertension can occur with a normal platelet count, but it is even more likely when the platelet count starts to fall. Thus, an upper endoscopy to screen for esophageal varices is recommended in this patient even though she is not cirrhotic (PBC without the "C").

Surveillance for hepatocellular carcinoma is not recommended in PBC in the absence of cirrhosis. This patient should, however, undergo bone mineral densitometry testing. Osteoporosis occurs in up to one third of patients with PBC. The etiology of osteoporosis in PBC is not entirely clear; sometimes it occurs from vitamin D deficiency resulting from fat malabsorption, which tends to occur late in the disease course. Nonetheless, all patients with PBC should receive supplemental calcium (at least 1200 mg per day) and vitamin D (at least 800 IU per day). The replacement dose of vitamin D is much higher for those with a deficiency in this vitamin (which can be determined by checking levels of 25-hydroxyvitamin D). Osteoporosis is usually asymptomatic and is not associated with any particular laboratory abnormalities. Therefore, bone mineral densitometry should be performed upon diagnosis and at periodic intervals thereafter (eg, every 2 to 3 years). If patients are osteoporotic, then bisphosphonate therapy should be considered.

About 20% of PBC patients develop autoimmune-related hypothyroidism. In fact, thyroid disease can be detected several years before the PBC diagnosis is made. Thus, a TSH level should be checked on this patient as well. Identification and treatment of hypothyroidism can help reverse many signs and symptoms, including the neurologic and depressive symptoms that can often be confused with encephalopathy in patients with late-stage PBC. Sicca syndrome (which can be part of Sjögren's syndrome and includes dryness of the mouth [xerostomia], eyes [xerophthalmia], and vagina) and CREST syndrome (Calcinosis, Raynaud's, Esophageal dysfunction, Sclerodactyly, Telangiectasias) are more commonly found in PBC patients than in controls. Keep this in mind when autoimmune diseases present on exam. A patient with severe reflux symptoms with CREST syndrome, for example, may have an abnormal ALP, which would suggest the possibility of PBC.

Most patients with PBC also have hyperlipidemia. Yet despite this comorbidity, PBC patients are not at increased risk for atherosclerosis or cardiovascular events in the early disease course, probably because the HDL is typically high. However, LDL may increase in the late stages with a lowering of the HDL. You should check a lipid profile and consider lipid-lowering agents if the patient has risk factors or symptoms of coronary artery disease.

The patient in this vignette is on the correct dose of ursodeoxycholic acid at 13 to 15 mg/kg/day, which has been proven to delay the progression to end-stage disease, delay the need for liver transplantation, and increase survival. Higher doses of ursodeoxycholic acid do not have incremental efficacy compared with the 13 to 15 mg/kg/day dose. Unfortunately, no other single therapy has been consistently found to be helpful to delay the progression of this disease.

PBC has among the best survival rates after liver transplantation with more than a 90% 1-year survival. Recurrence does happen, but it typically does not progress rapidly enough to require retransplantation.

Why Might This Be Tested? PBC is a "classic," slowly progressive liver disease with several interesting manifestations. You will see patients who have PBC in your office and you should know how to diagnose them, but you should also know how to manage these patients for the long term. Board examiners have started to emphasize outpatient management of chronic diseases, not simply diagnostic decision making early in the disease course. That makes PBC a good bet to show up on the exam.

Clinical Threshold Alert: A dose of 13 to 15 mg/kg/day is the target range for therapeutic ursodeoxycholic acid for the treatment of PBC.

Here's the Point!

PBC → **Think of nodular regenerative hyperplasia, osteoporosis, and hypothyroidism**

Vignettes 34 to 37: Mallory Body Potpourri

You've been hearing about Mallory bodies since you were in medical school (and especially if you trained at Boston City Hospital, where the famed Mallory Institute of Pathology resides). Anyway, you know that Mallory bodies occur in alcoholic liver disease, but they show up elsewhere, too. This section includes a series of mini-vignettes of patients with Mallory bodies found on liver biopsy. Your goal is to figure out the underlying diagnosis. What are Mallory bodies, anyway? What are they made of? These questions and more are addressed in the answer section.

34. A 68-year-old man with atrial fibrillation develops liver test abnormalities after starting a new medication. Liver biopsy reveals phospholipid-laden lysosomal lamellar bodies along with Mallory bodies.

35. A 46-year-old woman with pruritus, progressive jaundice, and an elevated ALP undergoes liver biopsy revealing Mallory bodies and granulomatous destruction of the bile ducts with infiltration by lymphocytes and plasma cells.

36. An 18-year-old man presents with acute hepatitis with elevated aminotransferases but with a depressed ALP and uric acid levels. After recovery, a liver biopsy reveals periportal inflammation, interface hepatitis, and Mallory bodies.

37. A 58-year-old woman with diabetes and hyperlipidemia is found to have abnormal liver tests in labs performed as part of a routine physical. Laboratory values included the following: AST = 123, ALT = 159, ALP = 126, total bilirubin = 1.3. She consumes less than 30 g of alcohol per week. Liver biopsy reveals steatosis, lobular inflammation, ballooning hepatocytes, and Mallory bodies.

Vignettes 34 to 37: Answers

Mallory bodies are cytoplasmic inclusions within hepatocytes that are composed of cytokeratin intermediate filaments and ubiquitins, which are small regulatory proteins that are ubiquitously expressed in eukaryotes (hence the name ubiquitin). Mallory bodies have a characteristic "twisted rope" appearance on light microscopy (Figure 34-1). Although they are most common in alcoholic hepatitis, where they have a prevalence of around 65%, they are also found in a variety of other conditions, as described in the answers that follow.

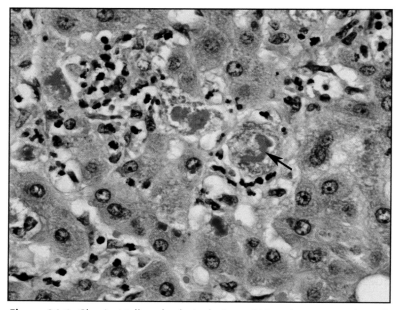

Figure 34-1. Classic Mallory body inclusion within a hepatocyte (arrow). The Mallory body has a characteristic twisted-rope appearance. This image reveals the inclusion within a ballooning hepatocyte, which is characteristic of both alcoholic and nonalcoholic fatty liver disease. (Reprinted with permission of Charles Lassman, MD, UCLA Medical Center.)

34. This is amiodarone toxicity. Refer to Vignette 15 for more details.

Here's the Point!

> Phospholipid-laden lysosomal lamellar bodies + Mallory bodies =
> Amiodarone toxicity

35. This is primary biliary cirrhosis. PBC is discussed in more detail in Vignette 33 and elsewhere, but the short story here is that Mallory bodies can be found in up to one quarter of liver biopsies from patients with PBC. If we had said the patient was positive for the antimitochondrial antibody (AMA), this exercise would have been too easy! AMA is positive in 95% of cases of PBC but can be negative on occasion, which is when a liver biopsy is typically useful. The natural history of PBC features 4 histologic stages. Stage 1, called the "portal stage," is marked by granulomatous destruction of the bile ductules. This is called a "florid duct lesion," which is a Board buzzword you should remember. The duct damage is accompanied by lymphocytic and plasma cell infiltration of the portal tracts (thus the "portal stage" designation of stage 1). In stage 2, called the "peri-portal stage," there is loss of the bile ducts (also called "ductopenia") along with extension of the inflammation to the periportal areas. In stage 3, there is septal fibrosis between adjacent portal tracts, and in stage 4, this organizes into cir-rhosis. Mallory bodies can be found throughout these stages. Figure 35-1 reveals a characteristic micrograph of PBC with granulomatous infiltration of the bile ducts and a florid duct lesion. It's important to remember that Mallory bodies can occur in PBC, but it's even more important to remember the granulomatous duct destruction of PBC, since that is a buzzword.

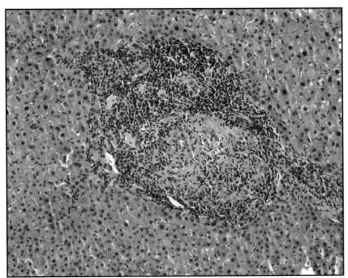

Figure 35-1. Micrograph of primary biliary cirrhosis with granu-lomatous infiltration of the bile ducts and a florid duct lesion. (Reprinted with permission of Charles Lassman, MD, UCLA Medical Center.)

Here's the Point!

Florid granulomatous duct lesion + Mallory bodies = PBC

36. This is Wilson disease. WD was discussed previously in more detail in Vignette 12, but for now let us review a few pearls about this condition (you can't go over WD enough). WD is an autosomal recessive condition marked by inadequate excretion of hepatic copper into the bile ducts (resulting from absent or reduced function of a gene called ATP7B—props to you if you can memorize that!). Bad things happen when copper builds up in the liver and blood. Liver manifestations include acute hepatitis, as occurred here, acute liver failure, and chronic disease marked by fibrosis and ultimately cirrhosis. In its earlier form, the liver biopsy reveals periportal inflammation, interface hepatitis, and bridging fibrosis. Mallory bodies are found in 25% to 50% of patients.

While we are on the topic of WD, here are the top 10 championship-level, clinically useful factlets to know (in no particular order):

- The acute hepatitis and acute liver failure phases of WD are often marked by an abrupt *hemolytic anemia.*

- *Low* ALP levels (not high ones) and low serum uric acid levels may occur in symptomatic liver or neurologic disease due to Fanconi syndrome of the proximal renal tubules.

- *WD happens in young people,* so if a Board question features a patient over 60 years of age, it's essentially incompatible with WD—don't be fooled.

- The presence of *neurologic findings is almost synonymous with cirrhosis*—it's very unusual to have neurologic findings in the absence of cirrhosis.

- Kayser-Fleischer (KF) rings occur from deposition of copper in the *Descemet's membrane* of the inner cornea, whereas the characteristic "sunflower cataract" is from copper deposition in the *lens capsule.*

- In the setting of classic neurologic symptoms from deposition of copper in the basal ganglia (eg, dystonia, chorea, dysarthria, Parkinsonian features), the presence of KF rings on slit-lamp examination is pathognomonic for WD, but the absence of KF rings with neurologic symptoms nearly excludes WD (ie, *high negative predictive value of absent KF rings when there are neurologic symptoms*).

- Although 95% of patients with WD have depressed serum ceruloplasmin levels (<20 mg/dL) and 85% have elevated urine copper excretion (>100 mcg/24 hrs), *low ceruloplasmin and high urine copper are sensitive but not entirely specific* for WD, because both are seen in some asymptomatic heterozygotes, among other conditions.

- The gold standard for diagnosis remains *quantification of hepatic copper,* where a concentration above 250 mcg copper/g dry tissue is diagnostic of WD—yet copper distribution may be heterogeneous, so a negative study does not entirely rule out WD, but a positive study is diagnostic in the right clinical setting.

- It's vital to *screen first-degree family members* of affected individuals with slit-lamp examination and measurement of serum ceruloplasmin levels.

- Both *neurologic symptoms and liver tests may initially worsen after starting therapy* (more so with D-penicillamine than trientine), but subsequent improvement typically occurs within 6 months of starting therapy (ie, it takes a while for the medicine to work, so don't discontinue it if the symptoms initially worsen unless there is a serious side effect).

Here's the Point!

Hepatitis + Depressed ALP + Mallory bodies = Wilson disease

Here's the Point!

Know the "top 10" facts of Wilson disease—Go back and read them again!

37. This is nonalcoholic fatty liver disease. NAFLD is covered elsewhere in this book, but this is a good opportunity to review some key facts about this astonishingly prevalent and important condition. By now you probably know that NAFLD is part of the metabolic syndrome, so it's commonly coupled with diabetes, hyperlipidemia, and of course obesity. A full accounting of NAFLD's pathophysiology is outside the scope of this book, but the quick and dirty point is that the metabolic syndrome predisposes to NAFLD through insulin resistance; this results in the subsequent accumulation of fatty acids in hepatocytes. When coupled with a "second hit" of oxidative stress, some people develop steatohepatitis and beyond. NAFLD is generally defined as hepatic steatosis (with our without steatohepatitis) exceeding 5% to 10% of the liver mass in the absence of significant alcohol consumption. How much alcohol can a patient consume and still be counted as having NAFLD? That is somewhat debatable, but a very conservative rule is less than 40 g per week, which isn't much. Recall from Vignette 26 that a standard alcoholic drink contains roughly 12 g of ethanol, so this rule means the patient has fewer than 4 drinks per week. Furthermore, in NAFLD the AST:ALT ratio is usually less than 1, in contrast to the typical 2:1 ratio in alcoholic hepatitis.

The liver biopsy in NAFLD depends on the grade of the disease, as follows: Grade 1 is basically steatosis alone without much inflammation; grade 2 is steatosis with lobular inflammation and ballooning hepatocytes but not much portal inflammation (Figure 37-1); grade 3 is steatosis, lobular inflammation, ballooning hepatocytes, plus portal inflammation. Of note, the diagnosis of nonalcoholic steatohepatitis, or NASH, which lies in the spectrum of NAFLD, is confirmed within these grades not only by the neutrophilic infiltration and hepatocyte ballooning, but also with the development of "chicken-wire" fibrosis (Figure 37-2). Mallory bodies can be seen throughout these various stages, but especially in more advanced stages.

Figure 37-1. Ballooning degeneration with fatty infiltration in NASH. (Reprinted with permission of Alton B. Farris, MD, Emory University.)

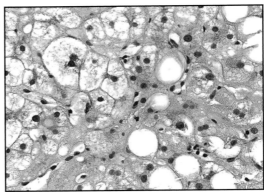

Figure 37-2. Nonalcoholic steatohepatitis with evidence of "chicken-wire" fibrosis investing the liver parenchyma on trichrome staining. The blue fibrous strands course between the ballooning hepatocytes in this advanced stage of disease. (Reprinted with permission of Charles Lassman, MD, UCLA Medical Center.)

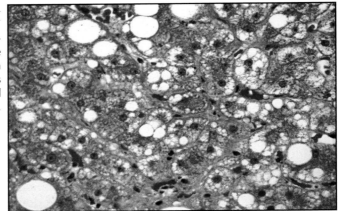

Here's the Point!

Metabolic syndrome + Low AST:ALT ratio + Mallory bodies = NAFLD

Vignette 38: Cough and Abdominal Pain

A 39-year-old man returns from a mission trip to rural Brazil. He has not been feeling well for the past 2 weeks. He has developed progressive symptoms of fever, right upper quadrant discomfort, right shoulder pain with inspiration, and coughing. He also reports fatigue for the past week without jaundice or weight loss. There has been no diarrhea or vomiting. He was not ill and had no medical problems while he was in Brazil for the past 6 months. Laboratory tests now reveal the following: WBC = 14 with left shift and 0% eosinophils, hemoglobin = 12.9, platelets = 290, total bilirubin = 1.1, ALP = 238, AST = 68, ALT = 80, albumin = 3.4, creatinine = 1.0, and INR = 1.0. Chest radiograph is remarkable for an elevated right hemidiaphragm. An abdominal CT scan is performed, shown in Figure 38-1.

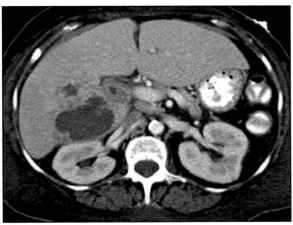

Figure 38-1. Abdominal CT for the patient in Vignette 38. (Reprinted with permission of Barbara Kadell, MD, UCLA Medical Center.)

▸ **What is the diagnosis?**

▸ **What do you do about it now?**

Vignette 38: Answer

This is an amebic liver abscess, which is the most common extraintestinal manifestation of amebiasis. The CT scan reveals a large, round, low-attenuation lesion with an enhancing rim measuring 6 cm in the right hepatic lobe. Although not seen in this image, right hemidiaphragm elevation is seen on chest X-ray (seen in about half of patients with amebic liver abscess). By the way, "right hemidiaphragm elevation" is a Board buzzword that often means "amebic liver abscess." For the patient in the case presented here, the next step is to perform serum testing for amebiasis, which will be positive about 95% of the time after 1 week of illness in a previously unexposed patient. Thus, serologic testing would be the best way to clinch the diagnosis. Aspiration, which carries a risk for subcapsular peritonitis, would not be a good idea and is not required for either diagnosis or routine treatment. In uncomplicated abscesses, antiamebic therapy alone is as effective as the combination of aspiration and antiamebic therapy. However, there are certain instances, as shown in Table 38-1, where aspiration or drainage of amebic liver abscesses is indicated (eg, when there is risk for imminent rupture or when a pyogenic abscess needs to be excluded). In these situations, close monitoring of the patient is critical, since rupture of the abscess with extension into the peritoneum, pleural cavity, or pericardium (which can occur with left lobe abscess) can be disastrous and requires emergent surgical therapy. Thankfully, most amebic abscesses occur in the right lobe, are solitary, and respond well to anti-amebic therapy with an ~1% mortality. When aspiration is performed, it might yield the classic "anchovy paste" substance; this is a chocolate-colored fluid composed of an admixture of blood and liver tissue (usually without visualization of the trophozoites on microscopy). We've never seen anchovy paste before, actually, so we'll just have to take their word for it.

This intestinal parasitic infection begins with ingestion (via the fecal-oral route) of contaminated water or food containing *Entamoeba histolytica* cysts. Excystation occurs in the intestinal lumen, where trophozoites can form new cysts in the mucin layer, resulting in an asymptomatic infection. This propagates the infectious cycle as the cysts are passed in stool. However, the trophozoites can occasionally invade the colonic lumen, causing an inflammatory response and the classic "flask-shaped" ulcerations, and extraintestinal spread can allow passage to the liver and other sites. Surprisingly, an antecedent diarrheal illness is not common and stool studies are typically negative in patients with amebic liver abscess. Leukocytosis without eosinophilia and an elevated ALP are common with an uncomplicated amebic liver abscess. However, hypoalbuminemia and elevated bilirubin are independent risk factors for increased mortality. The

Table 38-1.

INDICATIONS FOR ASPIRATION OR DRAINAGE OF SOLITARY AMEBIC LIVER ABSCESS

1. Lack of clinical improvement within 3 to 5 days
2. Seronegative abscess
3. Left lobe abscess
4. Thin rim of tissue (<1 cm) surrounding large abscess

abscess typically responds well to a 10-day course of metronidazole. Radiographic resolution can take several months despite clinical improvement. Even if stool studies are initially negative, a luminal amebicide (such as paromomycin) should be given after treatment of the liver abscess. Furthermore, follow-up stool specimens should be obtained upon completion of therapy to ensure against colonization and risk of recurrence. Unfortunately, infection does not confer immunity. Therefore, reinfection and recurrence of amebiasis are possible. Amebiasis is most often encountered in the United States in people who have traveled to tropical regions of Central and South America, southern Asia, and Africa.

It's important to distinguish amebic from pyogenic liver abscesses. Although pyogenic abscesses can appear radiographically similar to amebic abscesses, they can be distinguished clinically and radiographically in several ways. Unlike amebic abscesses, pyogenic liver abscesses typically derive from an intra-abdominal source of infection (such as appendicitis, diverticulitis, or cholangitis) or are secondary infections of underlying inflammatory bowel disease or malignancy. Pyogenic abscesses are often multiple and caused by bacterial seeding through the portal venous system, which feeds the liver with the bacteria. Therefore, unlike most amebic liver abscesses, they do require aspiration for diagnosis to guide antibiotic therapy, in addition to drainage and/or surgical therapy. In most circumstances, pyogenic liver abscesses also tend to occur in older patients, and have a slower recovery and worse prognosis than amebic liver abscesses. Table 38-2 summarizes the differences between pyogenic and amebic liver abscesses. Be sure that you don't confuse either of these with echinococcal cysts, which are something altogether different (more to come on that)!

Why Might This Be Tested? With increased globalization and without an effective vaccination, amebiasis tends to be commonly found in travelers to endemic regions. You should be able to recognize how this type of abscess differs clinically from pyogenic liver abscesses. Moreover, the luminal-liver correlations provide fodder for GI Board exam questions.

Table 38-2.		
AMEBIC VERSUS PYOGENIC LIVER ABSCESSES		
Characteristic	*Amebic Abscesses*	*Pyogenic Abscesses*
Typical number of lesions	Single	Multiple
Gender	Male predominance	Equal
Historical association	Traveler	Abdominal infection
Biliary involvement	Sterile	Infection common
Clinical response to therapy	Faster	Slower
Overall prognosis	Better	Worse

Here's the Point!

Right-lobe abscess + Right hemidiaphragm elevation + Recent travel = Amebic liver abscess (aspiration usually not mandatory)

Vignette 39: Ascites and Painful Gynecomastia

A 63-year-old man with alcoholic cirrhosis is started on 40 mg of furosemide and 100 mg of spironolactone once daily for control of ascites. Along with sodium restriction, the diuretics provide a good therapeutic response. A random urine Na is 25 mmol/L, and urine K is 8 mmol/L. Relevant serum laboratories include the following: Na = 135, K = 3.9, creatinine = 1.4. However, the patient reports painful gynecomastia after several weeks of receiving therapy.

▶ **What is the next therapeutic step?**

▶ **What if that step fails?**

Vignette 39: *Answer*

This is spironolactone-induced gynecomastia. Painful gynecomastia, or mastalgia, is one of the most common side effects of spironolactone in patients with cirrhosis. The decision about whether to discontinue spironolactone should be based on a determination of how effective the therapy for ascites has been, how severe the mastalgia really is, and whether the gynecomastia can be effectively treated while maintaining spironolactone on board. We will address this in a moment.

First, though, this is a good opportunity to review some time-tested pearls of wisdom regarding ascites management in cirrhosis. This is a big topic—much bigger than we can cover here—but the following are some of the high-yield facts.

The cornerstone of treatment in ascites is strict sodium restriction—not diuretics (although diuretics come in a close second). Patients should restrict their daily sodium to 2 g (88 mmol) or less. Of note, strict fluid restriction is generally not indicated in cirrhosis. This point seems perennially lost on inpatient teams who place a knee-jerk order to strictly limit fluids, especially when the sodium is a bit low. Fluid restriction certainly has a role when sodium gets really low in cirrhosis, but the general approach is to restrict sodium for managing cirrhotic ascites, not to strictly limit fluids.

Regarding diuretics, the usual approach is to begin with furosemide 40 mg and spironolactone 100 mg, both once daily. Split dosing is not necessary for these drugs in the management of ascites. This ratio of 40:100 is optimal to maintain normokalemia, since furosemide leads to hypokalemia, and spironolactone causes hyperkalemia. If the 40:100 ratio doesn't work, then move next to 80:200, and so forth, until you reach a maximum of 160:400. If that doesn't work (and assuming the patient is somewhat compliant with sodium restriction), then the patient has diuretic-resistant refractory ascites. The term *refractory ascites* is reserved for patients who have persistent ascites despite maximum diuretic therapy and sodium restriction (diuretic-resistant), or who have persistent ascites and can no longer tolerate diuretic therapy due to the side effects (diuretic-intractable; eg, if there is dose-limiting hyponatremia, azotemia, or renal insufficiency).

Along the way it's useful to check a random urine sodium level. The goal of diuretic therapy is to induce natriuresis, defined by a urine sodium exceeding 10 mmol/L; a urine sodium below this threshold suggests insufficient natriuresis, which is common in cirrhosis due to systemic vasodilation and upregulation of the renin and angiotensin. This process leads to release of antidiuretic hormone (ADH) with subsequent reabsorption of sodium and free water. In theory, a 24-hour urine collection is superior to a spot urine. The goal of diuretic therapy is to have more than 78 mEq/day of sodium in the 24-hour collection. But collecting a 24-hour urine is onerous and time-consuming, so most people use the random urine sodium as a barometer of whether there is adequate natriuresis. The ratio of urine Na to K has also been evaluated, and a ratio >1.0 (ie, more Na than K) is strongly predictive of >78 mEq/day of sodium in a 24-hour collection.

So, in this patient, things were going well until the gynecomastia. All it took was a starting dose of furosemide and spironolactone in the 40:100 ratio to induce adequate natriuresis (based on urine Na and urine Na:K ratio) and achieve a good clinical effect. Because furosemide alone is often inadequate for treating ascites in decompensated cirrhosis and can cause dangerous hypokalemia, the decision to discontinue spironolactone is not straightforward. The decision is further complicated by the fact that the traditional replacement for spironolactone, amiloride (another distal tubule agent), is less effective. If the mastalgia is enough to impact quality of life, then you can switch to amiloride at doses of 5 to 20 mg daily. If that doesn't work, then you can consider adding tamoxifen 20 mg twice daily to the aldactone. Randomized controlled trial data reveal that tamoxifen is highly effective and well tolerated for combating the spironolactone-induced gynecomastia.

Why Might This Be Tested? Ascites is a great topic for the GI Board exam because it's something everyone should know. But the GI exam is different from the ABIM internal medicine exam because the level of detail is greater and the expectation for knowledge is higher. So the exam might ask you to interpret a serum–ascites albumin gradient (SAAG), for example, but most everyone knows that already. It gets harder when the exam asks detailed management questions about rare but real problems, like mastalgia from spironolactone, or interpreting urine sodium levels.

Clinical Threshold Alert: If a patient on diuretics has <10 mmol/L of urine sodium on a random spot urine, or <78 mEq/day of sodium over 24 hours, then there is inadequate natriuresis and the diuretics should be further optimized. The same applies if the ratio of urine Na:K is less than 1.0.

Here's the Point!

Spironolactone can cause painful gynecomastia. If that happens, you can switch to amiloride or consider adding tamoxifen.

Vignette 40: An Unusual Case of Hepatitis

You are consulted to evaluate a patient in order to assist with the diagnosis of new-onset hepatitis. The patient is a 38-year-old Latino man who works as a chef in a local restaurant. Three days prior to admission, he developed chills, fever, and abdominal discomfort. He reported to his primary care doctor, who found that the patient was febrile (temperature = 101.2°F), had a pulse of 62, and had a blood pressure of 108/70. Outpatient laboratories included an AST of 192 and an ALT of 220. He was subsequently admitted for further evaluation of possible hepatitis.

On exam now he is febrile (temperature = 103.4°F) with a pulse of 66 and a blood pressure of 110/68. There is no orthostatic hypotension. Skin exam reveals faint, diffuse, salmon-colored macules across the trunk. He is not jaundiced, and there are no stigmata of chronic liver disease. He has diffuse tenderness in all quadrants with voluntary guarding but no rebound tenderness. Rectal exam reveals brown stool. Laboratories now include the following: hemoglobin = 10.6, WBC = 18.3 (90% PMNs), platelets = 288, amylase = 12, lipase = 15, ESR = 9, CRP <1.0, AST = 212, ALT = 246, LDH = 182. ALP = 204, total bilirubin = 1.8, INR = 1.1, albumin = 3.4.

▶ *What is the most likely diagnosis?*

▶ *Why?*

Vignette 40: Answer

This is typhoid fever from infection with either *Salmonella typhi* or *Salmonella paratyphi*. Typhoid fever is a classic Board-type condition because it can easily mimic other acute intra-abdominal processes. Plus, it can cause hepatitis and can easily be confused with viral hepatitis.

Typhoid fever usually begins within 7 to 21 days after ingestion of the culprit organism. It's rarely encountered in the United States and is most commonly contracted from ingestion of contaminated food or water in foreign countries (especially in those who neglected to get vaccinated for typhoid ahead of time). The prevalence of *S. typhi* and *S. paratyphi* is especially high in Nepal—a classic location for developing typhoid fever. This patient is not from Nepal, but had he just come back from Nepal with hepatitis, you would have to think about this. But, he is a chef, and you need to think about food contamination as a possible mode of transmission.

The condition usually begins with a complex of severe abdominal pain and "stepwise fevers," in which the fever curve follows a step-like pattern of progressive elevations. Another characteristic feature of the fever is a "temperature-pulse dissociation," in which the heart rate is bradycardic in relation to the fever. In this case, the pulse of 66 is quite low for such a high fever—even if this patient were an athlete. The abdominal pain of typhoid fever can be severe, and it's often in the right lower quadrant from underlying terminal ileitis or cecitis. In severe cases, the bowel can perforate, leading to a surgical emergency. In the second week of the illness the patient may develop so-called rose spots, which are faint salmon-colored macules across the trunk, as mentioned here.

The key for this vignette is that patients may also develop a hepatitis-like picture with elevated transaminases and bilirubin. The red herring in a Board exam would be to confuse this with simple viral hepatitis. Certainly hepatitis A is high on the differential for a chef coming in with a fever and biochemical hepatitis. But there are too many clues here to point away from simple viral hepatitis. The temperature-pulse dissociation is one clue; another is the presence of "rose spots." In addition, the ratio of ALT to LDH has been cited as a distinguishing feature, where a ratio of <4 is common in salmonella hepatitis, whereas a ratio of >4 to 5 is more common in acute viral hepatitis (see Vignette 1 as well). Data also reveal that compared to viral hepatitis, salmonella hepatitis is associated with higher peak fevers, higher ALP levels, and a higher white count with a left shift. The bottom line is that viral hepatitis can be clinically indistinguishable from salmonella hepatitis, but the biochemical patterns can help distinguish between them, especially when coupled with physical findings of relative bradycardia and characteristic skin rashes. Oh, and don't forget to treat the *Salmonella*, typically with a fluoroquinolone.

Why Might This Be Tested? Board examiners love anything that may affect the terminal ileum, and this condition is one of the classics. It's also full of Board buzzwords, like "temperature-pulse dissociation," "rose spots," and abdominal pain and fevers after being in Nepal. Finally, it affects both the intestines and the liver, so it can be "counted" in both bins as test-makers ensure sufficient coverage of all content frontiers. In short, it seems like a good condition to know about for the exam.

Here's the Point!

"Stepwise fever" + Temperature-pulse dissociation + "Rose spots" + Hepatitis
= Typhoid fever

Vignette 41: Liver Failure During a Marathon

A 38-year-old man was running a marathon on a hot day (82°F) when he collapsed at mile 18. Emergency medical technicians arrived to find the patient stuporous. Vital signs in the field were as follows: heart rate = 162, blood pressure = 98/62, respiratory rate = 22, O_2 saturation = 96%, temperature = 104.8°F. Cooling measures and intravenous fluids were initiated, and the patient was urgently transferred to the emergency department, where he arrived unconscious with a blood pressure of 102/70 and a rectal temperature of 103.6°F. Admission laboratories were as follows: AST = 78, ALT = 118, LDH = 451, ALP = 80, INR = 1.2, total bilirubin = 1.8, CK = 812, creatinine = 2.0, Na = 150, phosphate = 1.1. Over the next 24 hours he received intensive care with continued cooling measures and intravenous hydration. His mental status slowly improved, and he regained consciousness but remained drowsy. His blood pressure stabilized, and he was never hypotensive. The core temperatures normalized after 24 hours. By 48 hours, however, he became rapidly jaundiced and was found to have the following laboratories: AST = 1004, ALT = 1200, LDH = 899, ALP = 120, INR = 2.9, total bilirubin = 16.4, CK = 1002, creatinine = 1.6, Na = 139, phosphate = 1.1, AFP = 10.2.

▶ **What happened here?**

▶ **How can these specific lab values assist in determining prognosis?**

Vignette 41: Answer

This is acute liver failure resulting from exertional heat stroke (EHS). EHS is a diagnosis well known to paramedics and emergency medicine physicians, but we should know about it too because it can affect the liver. In fact, it can hammer the liver to the point of acute liver failure requiring transplantation. EHS occurs when environmental heat overcomes the body's ability to dissipate heat. This naturally leads to an increased core temperature, which, before long, precipitates a cascade of multiorgan damage. Cardiovascular collapse is the most common and feared complication of EHS, but liver damage is nearly universal as well. In most cases, hepatic injury is mild or moderate and associated with transient increases in the liver tests. But in some cases, the EHS can cause extensive hepatocellular injury, acute liver failure, and death. The injury is not necessarily from hypotension, as can be seen with ischemic hepatitis (although in both cases the LDH tends to be quite high and the ALT:LDH ratio low, as seen here), but from a variety of mechanisms including endotoxinemia (so called heat sepsis) and high blood concentrations of cytokines and acute-phase proteins.

The prognosis of acute liver failure in EHS can be poor—but not always. The good news is that many patients with this condition are young and otherwise healthy, so survival is often better than expected. In general, patients under 30 years of age have a better prognosis in acute liver failure (of any kind) than older patients do. And yes, being in your 30s is considered "old" when it comes to acute liver failure. This patient is 38, which makes him old enough for bad things to happen. But there are some bright spots in his biochemical profile. In particular, his AFP is elevated at 10.2. The AFP is usually employed to screen for hepatocellular cancer, but it has a prognostic role in acute liver failure as well. When the AFP is above 3.9 ng/mL the day after the ALT peaks, the likelihood of recovery is significantly improved. AFP is a surrogate marker for liver regeneration in the setting of acute liver failure. Another good sign is the hypophosphatemia. Low phosphate means the liver is kicking into gear and regenerating—a process that requires cellular uptake of phosphate to keep the machinery running under stress. So the combination of elevated AFP and low phosphate predicts a favorable prognosis in this otherwise very sick patient. Some people also measure factor V levels in acute liver failure because low factor V indicates a poor prognosis and diminished functional capacity of the remaining liver.

While we're on the topic of biochemical prognosticators in acute liver failure, it's worth remembering that rapid drops in aminotransferase levels are a bad thing. When you see the AST and ALT quickly rise and then quickly drop (sometimes to very low levels), it may suggest a "burnout" of the liver from overwhelming necrosis (see Vignette 1).

Why Might This Be Tested? Published case series of EHS reveal a surprisingly high prevalence of liver injury, yet this is not as widely appreciated as it probably should be. The severity of liver injury is often not appreciated until it's too late. Sometimes, these patients need a liver transplant, yet when the focus is on correcting body temperature, renal function, and cardiovascular function, it can become easy to forget about the liver. Once those systems are restored, the liver often remains dysfunctional, and the focus is only then fixated on the liver injury. The bottom line is that liver injury with EHS really happens and is often not realized until it's too late. The Board exam might also use a vignette like this as a way to see how well you know the biochemical prognosticators of acute liver failure.

Clinical Threshold Alert: If the AFP exceeds 3.9 ng/mL a day after the ALT peaks in acute liver failure, a favorable outcome is predicted.

Here's the Point!

**Really hot + Liver trouble = Hepatic injury from exertional heat stroke...
Watch out for acute liver failure!**

Here's the Point!

Favorable biochemical indicators in acute liver failure include:
- **Hypophosphatemia**
- **Elevated AFP**
- **Elevated factor V**

Vignette 42: Persistent Hypotension in Acute Liver Failure

A 42-year-old woman is admitted for management of acute liver failure from acetaminophen toxicity. She is admitted to the intensive care unit, where she is intubated and mechanically ventilated for advanced encephalopathy. After 72 hours of multidisciplinary management including treatment with N-acetylcysteine, she becomes progressively hypotensive, requiring vasopressor support. The hypotension continues for several days, during which time she is evaluated for cardiogenic shock and sepsis. Blood, urine, and sputum cultures are unremarkable, and cardiac evaluations are not consistent with a cardiogenic source of hypotension. An intracranial pressure (ICP) monitor is placed, which reveals an ICP of 10 mm Hg and a cerebral perfusion pressure (CPP) of 70 mm Hg. Despite fluid resuscitation and continued vasopressor support, the patient remains persistently hypotensive.

▶ *What should you look for next?*

Vignette 42: Answer

This is most likely adrenal insufficiency in the setting of acute liver failure. Did you get it? If not, you're not alone. It's easy to miss adrenal insufficiency as a cause of persistent hypotension in critically ill patients. But this is not just any critically ill patient—this patient has acute liver failure, and adrenal insufficiency is especially common in acute liver failure. One series from King's College in Britain (the source of the King's College Criteria described in Vignette 27) found that nearly two thirds of patients with acute liver failure have biochemical evidence of adrenal insufficiency, which is especially common in acetaminophen-induced liver failure, although it's certainly found in other etiologies as well. This is obviously important because adrenal insufficiency can mimic some of the hemodynamic anomalies seen in acute liver failure, including hyperdynamic cardiovascular collapse. The work from King's College has shown that patients with adrenal insufficiency are sicker, have more severe hemodynamic instability, are more likely to require liver transplantation, and are more likely to die compared to those without adrenal insufficiency. It remains unclear whether this is a cause-and-effect relationship or simply a marker of illness. But the key is to think about adrenal insufficiency early, test for it actively (typically with a cosyntropin stimulation test), and treat with IV corticosteroids on a timely basis. In fact, in this case it would be reasonable to empirically treat with IV steroids while awaiting the result of the stimulation test.

This vignette provides a good excuse to review ICP treatment goals in acute liver failure. In this case, the patient was evaluated for persistently elevated ICP despite hyperventilation and was found to have an ICP of 10 mm Hg and a CPP of 70 mm Hg. Both of those are right where you would want them to be. As an important aside, the need for ICP monitoring remains debatable—it's not necessarily standard of care to place ICP monitors in all patients with acute liver failure. The monitors themselves can cause problems, including intracranial bleeding and infection.

But assuming the ICP monitoring device is in and is working, it's good to remember a few numbers. The goal of therapy is to maintain ICP below 20 mm Hg. The CPP, in turn, should be higher than 50 to 60 mm Hg. The CPP is calculated by subtracting the ICP from the mean arterial pressure (MAP). So the higher the ICP, the lower the CPP, and the harder it is to get oxygenated blood to the brain—a bad combination. But if the ICP can remain low enough while the MAP is maintained at adequate levels, then the CPP will be higher and the patient's cerebral oxygenation will be improved. If the CPP falls and the ICP goes up, the usual first-line therapy is to start intravenous mannitol.

Why Might This Be Tested? Acute liver failure is eminently testable. And this vignette is great Board fodder because it simultaneously requires knowledge about acute liver failure and general internal medicine. Finally, if you miss this diagnosis, you might significantly worsen outcomes by failing to identify a treatable problem. Treating the problem may or may not save a life, but failing to make this diagnosis could definitely hurt a patient. Board examiners want to make sure that doesn't happen.

Clinical Threshold Alert: For elevated ICP in acute liver failure, the goal is to maintain ICP below 20 mm Hg and increase CPP above 50 to 60 mm Hg. And remember that CPP = MAP – ICP.

Here's the Point!

**Persistent unexplained hypotension in acute liver failure =
Think adrenal insufficiency**

Vignette 43: Abnormal Liver Tests (Yes, Again)

A 38-year-old Caucasian man is referred to you by his primary care provider for further evaluation of asymptomatic liver test elevations. He feels fine and does not have pruritus, fatigue, jaundice, or abdominal pain. Physical examination, BMI, and vital signs are all unremarkable. Laboratory tests show the following: ALT = 42, AST = 40, ALP = 180, GGT = 102, total bilirubin = 1.0, albumin = 4.2, creatinine = 1.0, INR = 1.0, WBC = 5.2, hemoglobin = 14.6, platelets = 259. You order a magnetic resonance cholangiopancreatography (MRCP), as shown in Figure 43-1. Liver biopsy is performed showing "fibrous obliteration of bile ducts with connective tissue replacement concentrically."

Figure 43-1. MRCP of the patient in Vignette 43. (Reprinted with permission of Barbara Kadell, MD, UCLA Medical Center.)

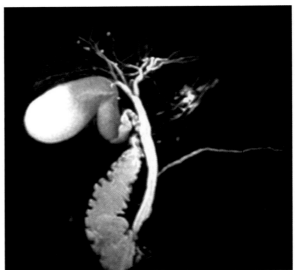

▶ *What is this?*

▶ *Are any other tests needed?*

Vignette 43: Answer

This is small-duct primary sclerosing cholangitis (PSC). Unlike in typical large-duct PSC, where liver biopsy is rarely needed since cholangiography is diagnostic, liver biopsy is essential in small-duct PSC since cholangiography is normal. So, if the MRCP in Figure 43-1 looked normal to you, you were right. Small-duct PSC can be diagnosed only with liver biopsy, not by cholangiography. In this case, the biopsy describes the classic "onion-skin" pattern of fibrosis, which clinches the diagnosis. That is, there is fibrous obliteration of the bile duct with concentric connective tissue replacement. About 5% of all patients with PSC have small-duct PSC, and these patients tend to have a more indolent disease course than patients with large-duct PSC; around 20% progress to large-duct disease and very few develop cholangiocarcinoma.

Even though the patient in this vignette is asymptomatic, a colonoscopy with biopsies should be undertaken to rule out concomitant inflammatory bowel disease (IBD), which is present in the majority of cases (see Vignette 93 for more on this).

While we are on the topic of PSC, let's focus on large-duct PSC for a moment. In patients with large-duct disease, especially in those without evidence of IBD, an IgG4 level should be checked. An elevation of IgG4 may signify an IgG4-associated cholangitis that can mimic PSC (and is sometimes associated with sclerosing of the pancreatic ducts and autoimmune pancreatitis). However, unlike PSC, IgG4-associated cholangitis can respond to a course of corticosteroids. Therefore, it's important to rule out IgG4-associated cholangitis in these patients.

Here are some interesting associations and tidbits related to PSC:

1. IBD is prevalent in the majority of patients with PSC; however, PSC is present in less than 10% of patients with IBD (more in Vignette 93).
2. IBD can occur de novo after liver transplantation for PSC.
3. PSC can occur de novo after proctocolectomy for ulcerative colitis (UC).
4. Patients with UC and PSC are at increased risk for colorectal neoplasia compared with patients with UC but not PSC. Furthermore, when colorectal neoplasia is found, it's in the right colon about 75% of the time. This stresses the importance of a full colonoscopy with a good bowel preparation regimen.
5. Ursodeoxycholic acid therapy is not effective to halt the progression of PSC and has increased side effects at the higher doses. Thus, it is not recommended routinely for PSC.
6. Cholangiocarcinoma occurs in about 10% of patients with PSC. However, as opposed to colorectal malignancy in UC, which tends to present well after the initial diagnosis of UC, cholangiocarcinoma is present within 1 year of the time of diagnosis of PSC in about half of the patients who develop it.
7. Gallbladder polyps in PSC are frequently malignant. Thus, cholecystectomy needs to be considered in PSC patients with significant gallbladder polyps.

Why Might This Be Tested? PSC and UC provide a great combination of gastroenterology and hepatology diseases occurring in the same patient. Furthermore, there are several associations with malignancy that are clinically relevant. This provides a perfect setup for the GI Board examiner. Expect to see some of this on the exam.

Here's the Point!

Small-duct PSC ⟶ Normal cholangiogram ⟶ Liver biopsy needed for diagnosis

PSC without IBD ⟶ Think of IgG4-associated cholangitis

And know the 7 PSC factoids listed in the discussion!

Vignette 44: Biliary Obstruction After Eating Dirt

A 21-year-old man is referred for ERCP in the setting of recurrent biliary colic. He emigrated from El Salvador 1 year ago and, upon careful questioning, acknowledged episodes of pica with eating dirt. He initially presented 8 months prior to this visit with classic biliary colic, and he similarly presented again 2 months before the current visit. He is now asymptomatic and does not report any GI symptoms, including fever, chills, nausea, vomiting, abdominal pain, or change in bowel habits. Physical examination is significant only for an enlarged liver. Labs include the following: hemoglobin = 15.7, AST = 92, ALT = 72, ALP = 113, total bilirubin = 1.8. Pre-ERCP ultrasonography revealed a liver span of 19.9 cm, diffuse fatty infiltration, tortuous tracks through the liver parenchyma, and a common bile duct dilated at 11 mm. There were multiple echogenic foci in the gallbladder and common bile duct. ERCP with sphincterotomy did not show stones, but instead revealed multiple flat parasites, as pictured in Figures 44-1 and 44-2.

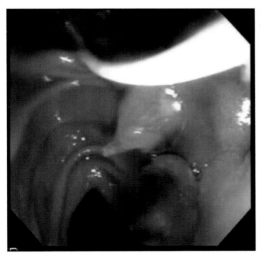

Figure 44-1. Flat parasites in the duodenum. (Reprinted with permission of Stanley Dea, MD, Olive-View UCLA Medical Center.)

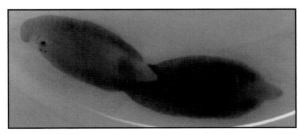

Figure 44-2. Flat parasites collected from patient after ERCP. (Reprinted with permission of Stanley Dea, MD, Olive-View UCLA Medical Center.)

▶ *What is the diagnosis?*
▶ *How should this be treated?*

Vignette 44: Answer

This is fascioliasis, which is an infection with either *Fasciola hepatica* or *Fasciola gigantica*. That's right, there is actually something called *Fasciola gigantica*. Yikes! This just shouldn't happen... but it does. There's nothing good about fascioliasis. Both *Fasciola hepatica* and *gigantica* are liver flukes, or trematodes, that occur all over the world. These flukes are most prevalent around sheep. In fact, they infect sheep and cause something called "liver rot." Like I said, there's just nothing good about this. Humans are an accidental intermediate host in the complex life cycle of these critters. Fascioliasis typically occurs in people who live in sheep-rearing communities most commonly in the temperate climates of Central America, South America, the Middle East, parts of Africa, and China. It even happens in the U.S. every so often, albeit rarely. Humans are usually infected by eating contaminated food products or drinking unboiled water contaminated by the parasites. In this particular case, the patient was not a sheep herder, but had a curious pica habit that led him to eat dirt. That probably caused him to become ill, but it's hard to say for certain.

Once these buggers are ingested, they eventually take up lodging in the biliary tree where they lay their nasty little eggs. These ultimately shed through the ampulla of Vater and are expelled in feces. They tend to hang out in water where they mature until a snail comes along and ingests them. They grow within the snail, get pooped out again, and then start hanging out on various aquatic vegetation. Eventually a sheep will come along and eat the vegetation and get sick. If a human eats these contaminated fresh water plants or if the water is directly consumed, then the infective forms are ingested (called *metacercariae*, if you really want to know). These next turn into the larvae in the duodenum (see Figures 44-1 and 44-2). It gets even nastier, because these larvae next eat through the wall of the small bowel and enter the peritoneum. From there, they head over to the liver and penetrate the capsule, where they proceed to burrow through the liver tissue. That's right—they can burrow right through your liver (kind of like a TIPS placement). Just look at the mouths of these things under microscopy (Figure 44-3). Once they penetrate the capsule, subcapsular hematoma can occur. The burrows themselves are large enough to show up as

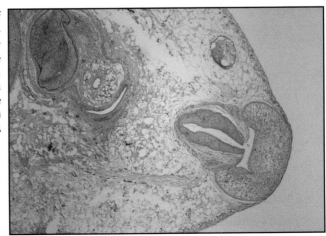

Figure 44-3. Histologic section of *Fasciola* parasite showing the mouth-like area. This parasite eats its way through the intestinal wall, into the peritoneum, through the liver capsule, and through the liver parenchyma before finally taking residence in the biliary tree. (Reprinted with permission of Stanley Dea, MD; Olive-View UCLA Medical Center.)

"tortuous tracks" on imaging. These tracks become necrotic, leading to liver rot. The trematodes then head over to the biliary tree where they start laying their eggs. They can totally plug up the biliary tree because they are so large—at least by parasite standards. (Not sure if they are really *gigantica*, but they are gigantica enough to plug up a biliary tree!) And then the cycle repeats itself. I mean, you've got to be kidding!

Treatment for fascioliasis is a little tricky because some of the usual therapies are not effective against this liver fluke. Specifically, praziquantel, mebendazole, and albendeazole don't seem to work. Nitazoxanide does have some efficacy, however, with a cure rate approaching 80%. In this case, the patient was treated with nitazoxanide 500 mg twice daily for 7 days and had complete resolution of symptoms. He may still be eating dirt, however.

Why Might This Be Tested? Clearly this is a rare infection in the United States, at least. But, it happens. Plus, we tend to focus too much on viral infections of the liver so it becomes easy to forget about the various nonviral infections that befall it. Board examiners may reserve the right to trailblaze off the viral infection highway and explore some less frequented, yet still important, liver infections. Other classic nonviral infections of the liver include pyogenic liver abscesses, amebic liver abscesses, schistosomiasis, clonorchis sinensis, and everyone's favorite—echinococcosis. Table 44-1 provides some board buzzwords you can remember to quickly sort out the diagnosis and treatment for the usual suspects. This table alone is probably enough to get you most of the way through questions about these infections.

Table 44-1.	
BOARD BUZZWORDS FOR LIVER PARASITES	
Board Buzzword/Association	**Associated Condition(s)**
Sheepherder	Fascioliasis, echinococcosis
Strong male predominance	Amebiasis
Serum sickness (aka Katayama fever)	Schistosomiasis
Solitary hepatic cyst of right lobe	Echinococcosis, amebiasis
Portal vein granulomas and fibrosis	Schistosomiasis
Hepatic abscess with elevation of right hemidiaphragm with adhesions obliterating the costophrenic angle	Amebiasis
Transverse myelitis	Schistosomiasis
Anaphylaxis after cystic rupture	Echinococcosis
Abscess filled with "anchovy paste"	Amebiasis
Epilepsy	Schistosomiasis
Smooth, round cyst with internal septations	Echinococcosis
Undercooked fish	Clonorchiasis
	(continued)

Table 44-1 (continued).	
BOARD BUZZWORDS FOR LIVER PARASITES	
Board Buzzword/Association	*Associated Condition(s)*
Portal hypertension without stigmata of chronic liver disease	Schistosomiasis
Gallstones	Clonorchiasis
Biliary ductal fibrosis	Clonorchiasis
Liver cyst with eggshell calcifications	Echinococcosis
Contaminated freshwater plants	Fascioliasis
Cyst filled with "hydatid sand"	Echinococcosis
Tortuous tracks in liver on CT	Fascioliasis
Tsetse fly	African trypanosomiasis (aka sleeping sickness)
Cyst surrounded by "daughter cysts"	Echinococcosis
Reduviid bug (aka kissing bug)	American trypanosomiasis (aka Chagas disease)
Sandfly	Leishmaniasis (kala-azar)

Here's the Point!

Sheepherder + Liver with "tortuous tracks" on CT + Biliary obstruction = Fascioliasis (usually from *F. hepatica*, less commonly from *F. gigantica*)

Vignettes 45 to 49: Hepatic Bruit Potpourri

Hepatic bruits. Have you ever really heard one? If you listen long enough to enough patients, you will hear one eventually. Of course, knowledge of hepatic bruits tends to be more valuable on Board exams than in real life, but it also makes for great roundsmanship to pick up a bruit. The following mini-vignettes describe patients in whom a hepatic bruit was auscultated. Try to figure out the most likely cause of the bruit in each vignette.

45. A patient is brought into the emergency department by paramedics after being found lying unconscious on a sidewalk. On exam, there are no stigmata of liver disease, but the patient is jaundiced and there is a hepatic bruit. The laboratories include an AST = 212 and an ALT = 89.

46. A patient with hepatitis B cirrhosis and HBsAg and HBeAg double positivity presents with progressive hepatic encephalopathy. Exam reveals a new hepatic bruit.

47. A patient presents with recurrent right upper quadrant abdominal pain. Physical exam reveals no stigmata of liver disease but a hepatic bruit. Ultrasound reveals a normal gallbladder and biliary tree, but there is a cystic mass in the gastroduodenal ligament between the pancreatic head and left liver lobe. A CT scan confirms this lesion and reveals vascular contrast enhancement within the cystic structure.

48. A patient with cirrhosis and progressive ascites develops prominent umbilical and periumbilical vessels followed by progressive improvement of the ascites. Auscultation over the abdominal vessels reveals a constant humming sound (okay, not quite a hepatic bruit, but a periumbilical bruit, so to speak).

49. A patient is stabbed in the abdomen. Exploratory laparotomy reveals liver lacerations, which are then sutured closed. The patient recovers from surgery and is discharged. He returns several weeks later with right upper quadrant pain. Physical exam reveals a continuous hepatic bruit and stool positive for occult blood.

Vignettes 45 to 49: Answers

45. This is acute alcoholic hepatitis (AH). Refer to Vignette 26 for much more on AH. In this case, AH is likely given the AST:ALT ratio exceeding 2:1 coupled with the patient being found unconscious (probably drunk). The point here is that patients with AH can present with a hepatic bruit on physical exam. The bruit probably results from an elevated hepatic artery diameter and increased arterial flow in the setting of acute AH. These findings can be seen on duplex Doppler ultrasound, although the diagnosis is usually clinched without the need for this test.

46. This is concerning for hepatocellular carcinoma (HCC). Patients with hepatitis B cirrhosis are at especially high risk for cancer, in general, so you always need to be on the lookout for HCC in this population. The risk is especially high in patients who are both HBsAg and HBeAg positive. Those with double positivity have a 60 times higher risk of developing HCC compared to patients who are double negative for HBsAg and HBeAg. Those who are positive for HBsAg alone are around 10 times more likely to develop HCC than patients who are double negative, which is still high, but it's the HBeAg positivity that really confers the major risk. This patient is double positive, so the risk of HCC is especially high. And HCC, in turn, is a hypervascular lesion that can sometimes generate a hepatic bruit on auscultation. Although this is not the usual way that HCC is identified, there are some instances when HCC is detected by auscultating a hepatic bruit. Another pearl of wisdom is that new-onset hepatic encephalopathy should also trigger a search for underlying HCC if there are no other obvious causes for the encephalopathy (see Vignette 11).

It's nearly impossible to overstate the epidemiologic importance of HCC. Whereas the incidence of cancer has been slowly dropping across most major cancer diagnoses, the same cannot be said for HCC. With the rising tide of patients with chronic hepatitis C and NAFLD, we are now witnessing a tidal wave of new HCC diagnoses. HCC is the third leading cause of cancer death and the fourth most prevalent malignancy worldwide. According to the World Health Organization, over 500,000 people globally die each year from primary liver cancer. So you can rest assured that HCC will be on the Board exam—if it isn't, then the examiners are not doing their job.

47. This is an extrahepatic hepatic artery aneurysm (HAA). Extrahepatic HAA most often occurs in the setting of atherosclerosis, but it also has been described with medial degeneration, trauma, and mycotic infection. Intrahepatic HAA, in contrast, is usually a false aneurysm resulting from trauma. Although less relevant for a general GI examination, anastomotic complications from orthotopic liver transplantation can also lead to HAA.

HAA can be very dangerous (perforation and exsanguination in up to 20% of patients), but it's hard to diagnose since most people are asymptomatic. Patients sometimes have symptoms that are biliary in nature, like this patient, who presented with recurrent right upper quadrant abdominal pain. Ultrasound imaging may demonstrate a cystic mass, although this can be mistaken for a tumor. Follow-up CT is more reliable for demonstrating the vascular contrast enhancement within an HAA (Figure 47-1). Extrahepatic HAA often occurs in the gastroduodenal ligament between the pancreatic head and the left liver lobe, as was seen here. This type of HAA is treated surgically, typically with proximal and distal ligation, since the gastroduodenal artery serves as a collateral vessel to help supply the liver. But an HAA that arises distal to the gastroduodenal artery requires a more extensive repair. When an HAA is intrahepatic, things get more difficult—in some cases partial liver resection is necessary to remove the aneurysm.

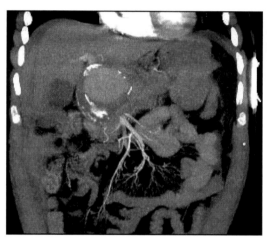

Figure 47-1. Hepatic artery aneurysm with calcifications appearing as a cyst-like structure near the porta hepatis. (Reprinted with permission of Barbara Kadell, MD, UCLA Medical Center.)

48. This is the Cruveilhier-Baumgarten murmur from an underlying spontaneous portosystemic shunt due to portal hypertension. This is the ultimate in roundsmanship—virtually every hepatologist asks unsuspecting students, residents, and fellows about this sign. In fact, they have been known to look at others in amazement if they don't know this eponym, almost as if the person didn't go to medical school. Although it's not really vital to know this sign, it's eminently testable. The Cruveilhier-Baumgarten murmur occurs when there is recanalization of the umbilical vein and reversal of blood flow from the liver into the abdominal veins, which can give rise to a caput medusae, or "Medusa's head." In some cases this coincides with improvement of the underlying ascites, likely because the new portosystemic shunt helps to mobilize fluid by bypassing the portal blockade.

49. This is a traumatic arteriovenous (AV) fistula, possibly between the hepatic artery and the portal vein. The vignette does not give you enough information to know for sure, and this could even be an HAA, as seen in Vignette 47. But the persistent symptoms several weeks after an operation suggest a persistent and previously unrecognized AV fistula from the trauma. Normally AV fistulas lead to high-output heart failure, but this is less common when the AV fistula is intrahepatic. Based on experiments in dogs going back to the 1960s, fistulas between the portal vein and hepatic artery are dampened by resistance in the surrounding hepatic sinusoids, so patients do not fall into heart failure the way they might with AV fistulas in other parts of the body. But they often do have persistent abdominal pain or discomfort, and they may even have low-grade hemobilia from leakage into the biliary system (as seen here). Treatment is usually to fix these surgically.

Vignette 50: Coffee and the Liver

Let's say you drink a lot of coffee.

...That's the whole vignette.

▶ *Does this habit protect you from liver problems?*
▶ *If so, which problems, and why?*

Vignette 50: Answer

There has been a lot of talk about the relationship between coffee consumption and liver disease—so much that it's now reasonable to expect a Board question on this topic. This relationship is more than an epidemiologic oddity at this point; data have been mounting for years that coffee consumption may be protective against certain forms of liver disease. Indeed, meta-analyses have looked at the protective benefits of coffee consumption in this regard.

The strongest data pertain to protection against hepatocellular cancer, in particular. Overall, drinking 2 cups of coffee per day is associated with a roughly 40% reduction in liver cancer compared to drinking less coffee. This protective effect is not only in those with pre-existing liver disease, such as cirrhosis, but even in those who do not have cirrhosis—although the benefits are larger in the former group (about 45% reduction in those with liver disease, and 30% in those without liver disease). There also seems to be a dose-response relationship between coffee consumption and hepatocellular cancer (ie, the more coffee you drink, the higher the protection). The protection is not just for liver cancer, but also for earlier forms of liver injury. Coffee consumption has been inversely associated with aminotransaminase levels in studies from around the world, with an especially strong benefit in those who drink a lot of coffee. So, coffee consumption appears to be protective against developing cirrhosis in the first place, even prior to developing liver cancer. In addition, recent data suggest that high levels of coffee consumption (more than 3 cups per day) improves virologic response to peginterferon plus ribavrin in patients with hepatitis C. Finally, there is evidence that coffee consumption can reduce the progression of disease in patients with chronic hepatitis C virus infection.

The way in which coffee might protect people from liver injury remains unclear. It seems to be more than the caffeine alone, although caffeine may be part of the story. The bottom line is that nobody really knows, so you would not need to know the mechanism for a Board exam.

You should, however, know that the relationship between coffee consumption and liver disease is an association, not a cause-and-effect relationship. Understanding the difference between causation and association is important. In fact, this is fair game for a Board exam, since the exam includes a variety of questions on study design, evidence-based medicine, and epidemiology. In order for something to be causal, several things need to line up, including the following: (1) There needs to be biologic plausibility for the relationship; (2) there should be a consistent association among many different studies with different populations and designs; (3) there should be a temporal relationship, such that the exposure comes first and the outcome follows; and (4) there should be a dose-response relationship, so that the more someone is exposed to the risk factor, the more likely he or she is to develop the outcome of interest. In the case of coffee and liver disease, there appears to be some biologic plausibility, the findings seem reproducible among many studies, and there is a dose-response relationship. However, there is not a clear temporal relationship—demonstrating that would ultimately require a prospective, randomized, controlled trial. It's also possible that the relationship is confounded such that patients with liver disease might end up drinking less coffee because of their illness—not that the coffee protected them. For now you should at least recognize that there is a pretty good case that coffee is somewhat protective against elevated aminotransferase levels, hepatitis C progression, cirrhosis, and even hepatocellular cancer.

Why Might This Be Tested? Liver cancer, in particular, is a hot topic. And the epidemiology of liver cancer is also increasingly important. Since coffee is now widely considered to be a protective factor for liver cancer, this epidemiologic observation is eminently testable.

Here's the Point!

Coffee consumption is epidemiologically protective against elevated AST/ALT, cirrhosis, and hepatocellular cancer.

Vignette 51: Mushroom Madness

A 51-year-old American woman developed colicky abdominal pain and watery diarrhea 1 day after eating a mushroom she found while hiking on vacation in Ireland. She nonetheless boarded a plane to return to the United States and developed progressive nausea and vomiting while en route. Upon arrival she reported to her local hospital, where she was found to be delirious, jaundiced, hypotensive, and tachycardic. Lab tests included the following: total bilirubin = 8.2, INR = 4.2, AST = 190, ALT = 210, albumin = 3.2, and creatinine = 2.1.

▶ **What happened here?**

▶ **How should this be treated?**

Vignette 51: Answer

This is acute liver failure from mushroom poisoning with *Amanita phalloides*. The *Amanita* mushroom, also known as the "death cap," is found across many parts of Europe, including Ireland (as in this case). In contrast, the death cap is not commonly found in the United States. All it takes is 30 g, or about half a normal mushroom cap, to kill an adult. The mushroom is full of toxins, including amatoxins and phallotoxins. These toxins inhibit RNA polymerase II, which ultimately shuts down the synthesis of essential proteins. The effect is most marked in the liver, since that is where the toxins are first encountered after ingestion. The toxins can also cause a hemolytic anemia and can often lead to kidney damage as well. When the toxicity is severe, acute liver failure and death can occur.

The treatment for *Amanita*-related liver failure is similar to the treatment for other forms of acute liver failure. In particular, it's important to screen for evidence of elevated intracranial pressure, monitor acid-base and renal status, ensure an intensive level of care, and triage for liver transplantation when necessary. It's also worth performing gastric lavage if the ingestion was known to be recent. Unfortunately, the patient typically presents days after the initial ingestion. For the Board exam, remember that these patients should also receive continuous infusions of penicillin G, although the mechanism of action remains unclear. In addition, extract of silymarin, or milk thistle, has been used successfully. The milk thistle extract is thought to prevent uptake of the amatoxins by the hepatocytes; it also may stimulate RNA polymerases, thereby kick-starting RNA synthesis and helping to reverse the effects of the *Amanita* toxins.

Why Might This Be Tested? Acute liver failure is eminently testable. So you should know acute liver failure 6 ways to Sunday, so to speak. This is just another in a long list of unusual presentations of acute liver failure. Moreover, it has a specific antidote that could be easily tested on an exam (milk thistle and penicillin G). Be prepared for unusual etiologies of acute liver failure, such as exertional heat stroke (Vignette 41), latent hepatitis B reactivated during immune reconstitution (Vignette 30), kava kava ingestion (Vignette 14), and so forth.

Here's the Point!

Mushroom ingestion + Acute liver failure = *Amanita* (death cap) poisoning.
Start penicillin G and silymarin (milk thistle extract).

Vignettes 52 to 55: Vitamin Power!

Vitamins are organic compounds that cannot be made by humans but are required as dietary nutrients to prevent metabolic disorders. Fat-soluble vitamin deficiencies are common in cholestatic liver disease, especially after the development of jaundice. It's important to know how to identify these vitamin deficiencies. The following mini-vignettes describe signs and symptoms of patients with end-stage cholestatic liver disease. For each, identify the culprit vitamin deficiency and specify the supplementation strategy.

52. Problems with balance while ambulating.

53. Difficulty driving at night.

54. Persistent bleeding after polypectomy.

55. Hip pain with osteopenia on DEXA scan.

Vignettes 52 to 55: Answers

52. This is vitamin E (tocopherol) deficiency, with classic symptoms of ataxia and gait disturbance. These patients can also have peripheral neuropathy and hyporeflexia. If you think about it, this scenario would also be typical for a case of overt hepatic encephalopathy, which highlights the importance of checking levels of vitamin E when you encounter neurologic symptoms like this in a patient with cholestatic liver disease. Vitamin E is an antioxidant and is responsible for the protection of cell membranes from oxidative damage. It's found in vegetable oils, meat, and eggs. Under normal conditions, we need just a touch of vitamin E to avoid neurologic sequelae from deficiency; only 15 mg (approximately 22 IU) is recommended on a daily basis. However, greater amounts are required for supplementation in vitamin E deficiency states (typically 1000 IU per day).

Here's the Point!

Cholestatic liver disease + Ataxia = Think about vitamin E deficiency

53. This is vitamin A (retinol) deficiency. A sophisticated people well ahead of their time, the ancient Egyptians fed liver to people with night blindness—pretty smart! More recently, we have learned that liver is an excellent food source for vitamin A. Retinol is also found in egg yolks, butter, and carrots. Other symptoms of vitamin A deficiency include hyperkeratosis and xerophthalmia with corneal and conjunctival xerosis. If a patient has symptoms of vitamin A deficiency, serum retinol levels should be checked. Levels less than 20 mcg/dL should prompt replacement of vitamin A. The recommended daily allowance of vitamin A is 900 mcg, or 3000 IU. Higher doses are needed in deficient states (typically 10,000 to 25,000 IU per day). However, care should be taken to avoid overdosing, because chronic toxicity can occur when over 50,000 IU are taken daily (see Vignette 21). This has been known to occur in some "health nuts" who take excessive amounts of vitamins, including vitamin A. Overdosing can lead to cirrhosis with liver biopsy showing Ito (fat-storing) cell hyperplasia with vacuoles.

Here's the Point!

Cholestatic liver disease + Night blindness = Think about vitamin A deficiency

54. This is vitamin K deficiency. Mucosal bleeding (which occurred after polypectomy here) and easy bruising are hallmarks of vitamin K deficiency. As you probably recall from medical school, vitamin K-dependent factors (II, VII, IX, X and protein C) are intricately involved in coagulation. Vitamin K is found in leafy vegetables and can also be produced by gut bacteria (which can be undermined by antibiotics). Thus, when you treat an infection in a patient with cirrhosis and you notice that the patient has a drastic increase in the MELD score, the increase may not necessarily be from hepatic deterioration. That's a great setup for a Board question—a patient with PBC who develops bleeding and an elevated INR after starting antibiotic therapy for hepatic encephalopathy. The elevated INR might simply be due to vitamin K deficiency, not from progression of the liver disease. Administration of 10 mg of vitamin K can often correct the INR and can be given through multiple routes of administration, depending on the clinical scenario.

Here's the Point!

**Patient with cirrhosis starts antibiotics and MELD peaks =
Think vitamin K deficiency**

55. This is vitamin D deficiency. It seems like everyone is vitamin D deficient these days. Well, not everyone—but vitamin D deficiency is much more common than most people realize. For the GI Board exam, remember that vitamin D deficiency is particularly common in inflammatory bowel disease and celiac sprue. Serum testing with measurement of the 25-hydroxyvitamin D level can aid in the diagnosis and treatment of these disorders with the goal of a 25-hydroxyvitamin D level of greater than 30 ng/mL. Vitamin D is found in fish, eggs, and certain mushrooms (but not the kind of mushroom featured in Vignette 51!). It is also manufactured by skin, provided there is adequate exposure to sunlight. Replacement can be given in various forms in high doses and then tapered to reach the desired level. However, in malabsorptive conditions, the patient may require 10,000 IU of vitamin D with high doses of calcium (up to 4000 mg). Prevention of osteoporosis and fractures is extremely important in these patients because disabling fractures and lack of mobility can limit candidacy for liver transplantation. Thus, bisphosphonate therapy should be considered in patients with osteopenia to prevent osteoporosis if other risk factors for fracture are present.

Here's the Point!

Cholestatic liver disease + Osteopenia = Think about vitamin D deficiency

Why Might This Be Tested? Vitamin deficiencies are Board review fodder, both for internal medicine and subspecialty Board examinations. While you may think it will be easy to spot some of these deficiencies in an exam question, sometimes the most obvious answer will not be at the top of your mind during the stress of an exam. So, it's good to review all of the fat-soluble vitamin deficiency states while preparing for the test. In clinical practice, these deficiencies can be diagnosed and treated readily by the observant physician.

Vignette 56: Fatigue and an Elevated Antinuclear Antibodies

A 32-year-old woman presents to her primary care physician with a chief complaint of progressive fatigue. She does not recall signs of icterus and has not experienced a recent viral illness. She drinks alcohol on occasion, reporting only 1 to 2 glasses of wine on weekends. She is not using any medications, does not report herbal exposures, and is not using illicit drugs. Her past medical history is unremarkable. On physical exam, there are no stigmata of chronic liver disease, there is no icterus and no jaundice, and the abdominal exam is normal. Laboratory tests reveal a normal blood count, INR = 1.0, total bilirubin = 1.2, albumin = 4.1, ALT = 206, AST = 189, and ALP = 151. Further laboratories reveal a negative HBsAg and negative anti-HCV antibody. Antinuclear antibodies (ANA) is elevated at 1:640 and AMA is elevated at 1:320. Anti-smooth muscle antibody (anti-SMA) is 1:40. Serum ferritin is 280, and ceruloplasmin levels are normal.

▶ *What is the most likely diagnosis?*
▶ *What might a liver biopsy reveal?*

Vignette 56: Answer

This is an overlap syndrome of autoimmune hepatitis (AIH) and PBC. AIH can present in both typical and atypical forms, and it can be a difficult diagnosis to pin down. The diagnostic dilemma is compounded by the fact that AIH sometimes overlaps with other conditions, namely PBC and PSC.

This gets even more confusing because the AIH-PBC overlap syndrome can come in 2 different forms. One form includes patients who are positive for AMA with histologic evidence of AIH but without histologic evidence of PBC. Some call this condition AMA-positive AIH. The clinical course and natural history of AMA-positive AIH are very similar to those of the pure, type 1 AIH. The second form of AIH-PBC overlap includes patients who are positive for ANA and/or anti-SMA with histologic evidence of PBC but without histologic evidence of AIH. This is often referred to as autoimmune cholangiopathy. Others think this is just AMA-negative PBC—not really an overlap syndrome.

The main thing to understand is that AIH and PBC, in particular, can overlap, and this can have both diagnostic and therapeutic implications. Around 10% to 15% of patients initially diagnosed with PBC end up having biochemical and/or histologic evidence of overlapping AIH. The converse is true as well—around the same percentage of patients with AIH demonstrate some evidence of comorbid PBC. Sometimes these disorders are found together at diagnosis, but oftentimes the natural history is that one disorder occurs first, and the other follows in time.

The patient in this vignette has a markedly elevated ANA and AMA, along with elevated aminotransferases and an elevated (but not too elevated) ALP. The anti-SMA is not particularly high. The histology is not described, but there are clear biochemical markers of both AIH and PBC. The picture is suggestive of AMA-positive AIH; it's less suggestive of autoimmune cholangiopathy. Since the natural history of AMA-positive AIH is similar to that of type 1 AIH, treatment should follow the usual AIH guidelines. In contrast, patients with autoimmune cholangiopathy, or AMA-negative PBC, should be treated with ursodeoxycholic acid (UDCA) and often glucocorticoids.

Why Might This Be Tested? You know that the Board exam will feature a number of questions about AIH, PBC, and PSC. But examiners will want to see if you know the next step, which is how to identify and manage common overlap syndromes across these conditions. The AIH-PBC overlap, in particular, is a good one to test since it has 2 different forms with different natural histories and treatment approaches. This can be confusing, and what better than a confusing area to cull the wheat from the chaff among test-takers?

Here's the Point!

ANA positive + AMA positive + Elevated aminotransferases = AMA-positive AIH

ANA positive + Anti-SMA positive + AMA negative + Elevated ALP = AMA-negative PBC, also known as autoimmune cholangiopathy

Vignette 57: Holy Pilgrimage

A 38-year-old woman, recently divorced, went to Surat, India, for a spiritual awakening to "find herself." She received the usual vaccinations from a travel clinic prior to leaving. She has just returned to the United States and discovered that she is 6 weeks pregnant. She was promptly referred to see you because of complaints of fatigue, fever, anorexia, jaundice, dark-colored urine, and light-colored stools for the past 2 weeks. Abdominal ultrasound is significant for hepatomegaly. Laboratory tests reveal the following: ALT = 2310, AST = 1640, LDH = 1290, total bilirubin = 3.2, WBC = 9.1, INR = 1.4, platelets = 160.

▶ **What is the most likely diagnosis?**

▶ **Can this be prevented?**

Vignette 57: Answer

This is hepatitis E virus (HEV) infection, which can be confirmed with an IgM anti-HEV titer. Like HAV infection, there is no need to call it "acute" since there is no chronic form of this infection. Travel to an endemic region should tip you off to this diagnosis. HEV was first recognized in India more than 30 years ago and is not endemic in the United States, but international travelers to Asia, Africa, Central America, and the Middle East could become infected. In fact, there was an outbreak in Surat (which is where one of the authors of this book was born) that was reportedly due to a contaminated drinking water pipeline. This was corrected and led to marked improvements in sanitation thereafter. The incubation period for HEV is approximately 1 to 2 months before the classic symptoms of jaundice, anorexia, nausea, abdominal pain, and fever are declared. Since acute viral hepatitis is the most common cause of jaundice in pregnancy, you should also check serologies for HAV, HBV, HCV, hepatitis D virus (HDV), Epstein-Barr virus (EBV), and cytomegalovirus (CMV). By the way, you should know that CMV hepatitis can give a distinct histological appearance with an "owl's eye" due to the surrounding halo of the intranuclear inclusion (Figure 57-1). HAV infection is less likely in this case since the patient should have been vaccinated against HAV at the travel clinic.

Similar to HAV infection, HEV is an RNA virus spread via the fecal-oral route and is generally self-limited. But HEV can be more severe than HAV infection with up to a 4% mortality rate, and among pregnant women in the third trimester, the mortality rate is a sobering 20%. Acute herpes simplex virus (HSV) hepatitis (Figure 57-2) also has a marked increase in mortality in pregnancy. Therefore, empiric treatment with acyclovir should be considered until the diagnosis is confirmed. In contrast, HAV does not have an increased mortality in pregnancy.

Treatment for HEV consists of supportive care with referral to a liver transplant center if severe. There are 4 classified genotypes of HEV, and epidemiologic studies are in progress to better understand the differences. Furthermore, a recombinant well-tolerated vaccine shows promise for the future. Prevention is

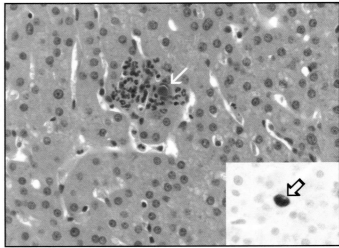

Figure 57-1. CMV hepatitis. An aggregate of neutrophils surrounds an infected hepatocyte [white arrow], containing an intranuclear inclusion with a surrounding halo, also known as an "owl's eye" inclusion. In the inset, CMV immunohistochemistry stains an infected hepatocyte [black open arrow], confirming the presence of CMV. (Reprinted with permission of Alton B. Farris, MD, Emory University.)

the key for now. International travelers should be wary of drinking water and/or ice of unknown purity and avoid uncooked seafood and unpeeled/uncooked fruits and vegetables that are not prepared by the traveler.

Why Might This Be Tested? There are more people traveling globally these days, leading to more infectious diseases coming home. We have said before that pregnancy is a favorite topic on Board exams; examiners especially like to include conditions for which there is a marked difference in pregnancy.

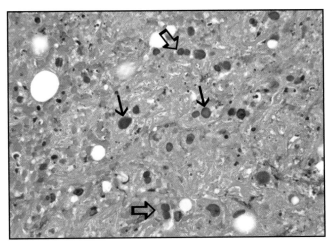

Figure 57-2. HSV hepatitis. The hepatic parenchyma shows extensive necrosis with scattered hepatocytes with glassy nuclear inclusions [arrows] and occasional multinucleated cells [open arrows] amidst the necrosis. (Reprinted with permission of Charles Lassman, MD, UCLA Medical Center.)

Here's the Point!

Traveler to Indian subcontinent with acute hepatitis → Think hepatitis E

Here's the Point!

HEV and HSV hepatitis → Increased mortality in pregnancy

Here's the Point!

Intranuclear "owl's eye" inclusions → Think CMV

Vignette 58: Big Liver Cysts

A 41-year-old pilot with autosomal-dominant polycystic kidney disease (ADPKD) presents to your office for initial consultation, having recently moved to your area. She brings her abdominal MRI taken last year for you to review (Figure 58-1). Although her kidney cysts have not been problematic, she has encountered persistent problems with innumerable, diffuse, large liver cysts, as pictured. She describes chronic pain and recurrent infections from these lesions despite having received fenestration procedures for palliation. She was told by her surgeon that resection was not feasible due to the diffuse nature of her large hepatic cysts. In fact, her condition has limited her mobility and she is no longer able to fly planes. She now presents to you with anorexia and early satiety with a resultant 50-pound unintentional weight loss over the past 6 months. Her BMI has fallen to 19. Laboratories include the following: ALT = 21, AST = 22, total bilirubin = 1.0, ALP = 110, albumin = 3.2, BUN = 7, creatinine = 0.6, INR = 1.0, WBC = 8.2, hemoglobin = 13.8, and platelets = 190. Due to her signs and symptoms and the concern for gastric malignancy, you perform an esophagogastroduodenoscopy (EGD), which is remarkable only for the finding in the esophagus shown in Figure 58-2.

Figure 58-1. T2-weighted abdominal MRI of this patient. (Reprinted with permission of Barbara Kadell, MD, UCLA Medical Center.)

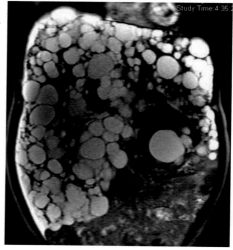

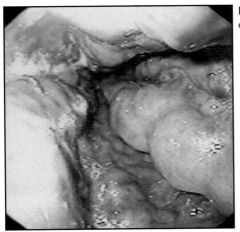

Figure 58-2. Esophageal lesions found on upper endoscopy.

▶ *What is going on here?*

▶ *What should you recommend for long-term treatment?*

Vignette 58: Answer

Those plump esophageal varices are indirectly due to autosomal-dominant polycystic kidney disease (ADPKD). Portal hypertension and the formation of esophageal varices can occur through a few different mechanisms in ADPKD, even in the absence of cirrhosis. The causes of noncirrhotic portal hypertension in ADPKD include portal vein compression by the massive hepatic cysts (thus, without ascites), hepatic vein or inferior vena cava compression by the massive hepatic cysts (thus, often with ascites), and congenital hepatic fibrosis in association with ADPKD (rare). Take a look at Vignette 3 for a refresher on portal hypertension.

Liver cysts are the most frequent extrarenal manifestation of ADPKD. The liver cysts tend to be more common in women than in men with ADPKD. Usually, liver cysts (with or without ADPKD association) do not pose much of a problem and rarely cause symptoms. As an aside, benign liver cysts in general (not associated with ADPKD) are also relatively common and occur in 4% of normals with a female predominance and increasing prevalence with advancing age. With benign liver cysts (whether ADPKD related or not), the liver parenchyma itself does not increase in size (therefore hepatic synthetic function is usually normal), but cystic enlargement can lead to massive hepatomegaly. This causes pain through stretch of the liver capsule and can also trigger other symptoms related to mechanical compression. The patient in this vignette had secondary gastric outlet obstruction from gastric compression, manifesting with early satiety and weight loss. In addition, compression of the venous system can lead to extrahepatic portal hypertension, as seen here. Unfortunately, this patient did not respond to cyst fenestration and was unable to undergo resection due to her diffusely large cysts.

Primary prophylaxis of variceal hemorrhage is indicated for this patient (see Vignette 13 for more on that). She should also be referred for consideration of liver transplantation before malnourishment poses a problem. Liver transplantation has its own set of risks, but the benefits would probably outweigh the risks in this particular case. If she is accepted onto a liver transplantation waiting list, the transplant center would need to appeal to UNOS for a higher MELD exception score, since her intrinsic MELD score (6) is normal. See Vignette 9 for more on MELD. So, this is a rare case where liver transplantation is reasonable even though there is no cirrhosis or liver synthetic dysfunction—seems like a nice setup for a Board question.

This particular patient should also be screened for an intracranial aneurysm, which occurs in 6% of patients with ADPKD without a family history of intracranial hemorrhage (16% with a family history). Screening for intracranial hemorrhage may not be appropriate for all patients with ADPKD. However, since the patient in this case is a pilot, it would be prudent to avoid the devastating consequences of an intracranial aneurysm rupture. Thus, screening with brain magnetic resonance angiography is indicated.

Why Might This Be Tested? Liver involvement is the most frequent extrarenal manifestation of ADPKD. The consequences of massive hepatomegaly can be difficult to manage. Liver transplantation can offer a last resort to select patients if other options do not help. The anatomic relationships of this condition are important to understand and fair game for the exam.

Here's the Point!

Massive liver cysts in ADPKD → Massive hepatomegaly → Portal hypertension and gastric outlet obstruction

Here's the Point!

Massive liver cysts + Intracranial aneurysm = Autosomal-dominant polycystic kidney disease (ADPKD)

Vignette 59: Autosomal-Dominant Polycystic Kidney Disease Case, Continued

The patient with ADPKD in Vignette 58 undergoes liver transplantation. She makes an excellent recovery, returns to flying (of course, after a screening brain MRA was negative), and enjoys spending time at the beach with her family. She has been doing well for 7 years after liver transplantation and is now 48 years old. However, today she comes into the emergency department with fever and sudden, severe, generalized abdominal pain with voluntary guarding and rebound tenderness on examination.

▶ *What known complication of ADPKD is this consistent with?*

▶ *What else does she need to worry about in the long term?*

Vignette 59: Answer

This is colonic perforation secondary to acute diverticulitis. Patients with ADPKD have increased frequency of diffuse colonic diverticulosis and complications related to diverticular disease. In addition, patients with ADPKD have an increased risk of abdominal wall hernias (45%) compared to controls (4%). Therefore, a patient with ADPKD who presents with abdominal pain needs evaluation for these possibilities as well as for renal cyst bleeding, infection, and/or rupture.

This vignette provides an opportunity to review some long-term complications of liver transplantation. Skin cancer is by far the most common malignancy that occurs de novo after transplantation. In particular, squamous cell carcinoma is the cancer with the highest incidence following liver transplantation. In contrast, basal cell carcinoma comprises 90% of skin cancers in immunocompetent patients. Thus, annual full-body skin examination is an extremely important preventive modality for routine health care maintenance in liver transplant recipients. Furthermore, it's important to advise patients to avoid prolonged sun exposure, especially during peak sun hours (9 AM until 4 PM), and to wear long sleeves and a hat when possible. Sunscreen is also important to help block both UV-A and UV-B radiation. In this case, the patient needs to know that prolonged sun exposure at the beach, although enjoyable, may increase her risk for developing skin cancer following liver transplantation.

Cardiovascular disease is also problematic in the long term after liver transplantation due to a combination of risk factors that develop. These include hypertension, hyperlipidemia, renal failure, and diabetes mellitus, which are in part due to immunosuppressive medications (especially calcineurin inhibitors, such as tacrolimus and cyclosporine). Chronic rejection is becoming much less of a problem. In fact, there has been a shift to using lower immunosuppression doses in the long term to decrease these secondary complications. Lowering immunosuppression should also help with reducing infections and malignancy, which are important causes of mortality in these patients. Furthermore, up to 40% of patients meet criteria for obesity within 1 year after transplantation, which contributes to cardiovascular complications over the long term as well. Vigilant management of these modifiable risk factors should help reduce long-term mortality.

Why Might This Be Tested? Survival has steadily increased following liver transplantation, which means that there are a larger number of post-transplant patients requiring long-term care and routine health care maintenance. Liver transplant centers are often returning these patients to the referring gastroenterologist for follow-up. It's important to recognize the possible complications that may arise so that preemptive therapy can be instituted.

Here's the Point!

Colonic diverticulosis and its complications are more common in ADPKD.

Here's the Point!

Squamous cell skin cancer is the most common malignancy after liver transplantation.

Here's the Point!

Calcineurin inhibitors increase risk for post-transplant hypertension, hyperlipidemia, diabetes, and renal failure.

Here's the Point!

Obesity is common following transplant and contributes to cardiovascular risk.

Vignettes 60 to 63: Low Alkaline Phosphatase Potpourri

High alkaline phosphatase (ALP) levels should conjure up a broad differential diagnosis. You can find a series of vignettes dealing with isolated elevated ALP in the first *Acing* book. Here we are focusing on the flip side: low ALP. The differential diagnosis of low ALP is relatively narrow, so what better excuse to tie together a few questions featuring this unusual lab finding? The following mini-vignettes describe patients with a low ALP. Try to figure out the most likely diagnosis for each one.

60. Ascites with SAAG >1.1, ascitic total protein >2.5, fatigue, constipation, hair changes, and a low ALP.

61. Developed gray hair early in life, now with dyspepsia, macrocytic anemia, and a low ALP.

62. A 20-year-old woman presents with acute hepatitis, hemolytic anemia, and a depressed ALP level.

63. A patient with Crohn's disease develops diarrhea and a scaling vesiculo-pustular plaque-like rash on the legs and face. The ALP is diminished.

Vignettes 60 to 63: Answers

60. This is hypothyroidism. On occasion, severe hypothyroidism can present with ascites and a low ALP. The ascites is typically characterized by a high ascitic total protein count and a high serum–ascites albumin gradient, or SAAG. An elevated SAAG is due to a transudative process such as cirrhotic ascites, acute liver failure, alcoholic hepatitis, or cardiac ascites from congestive heart failure. A SAAG <1.1 suggests an exudative process such as infection or malignancy. This case features a rare form of an elevated SAAG without portal hypertension and severe hypothyroidism (usually outright myxedema) due to an uncertain mechanism. The myxedema secondary to the hypothyroidism produces an elevated ascitic fluid total protein in combination with the high SAAG (similar to cardiac ascites). The low ALP observed in some patients with hypothyroidism is of unclear etiology. Some think the decreased ALP results from low serum zinc and magnesium levels in hypothyroidism. In any event, the ALP usually returns to normal with treatment. Refer to Figure 60-1 for a review of how to interpret the SAAG and ascitic fluid total protein.

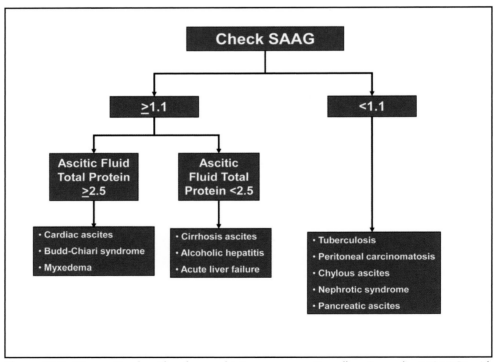

Figure 60-1. Diagnostic algorithm for combining serum–ascites albumin gradient (SAAG) with total protein of ascitic fluid.

Here's the Point!

Low ALP + High SAAG, High total protein ascites = Think hypothyroidism

61. This is pernicious anemia. Pernicious anemia is an autoimmune disorder marked by antiparietal cell antibodies, low intrinsic factor, and diminished vitamin B_{12} absorption with a macrocytic anemia. These patients often have comorbid autoimmunity. For example, early graying of the hair has been described in patients with pernicious anemia, which is probably an autoimmune phenomenon. The low ALP of pernicious anemia it thought to occur because osteoblast activity depends on cobalamin, and when there is cobalamin deficiency, bone metabolism is perturbed and ALP is diminished.

Here's the Point!

Low ALP + Macrocytosis + Early graying = Think pernicious anemia

62. This is acute Wilson disease (see Vignettes 12 and 36). There can be a marked depression in ALP levels in the acute phase of WD. The "Here's the Point!" for this vignette is the same as in Vignette 36—a point so pertinent we repeat it here.

Here's the Point!

Hepatitis + Depressed ALP + Mallory bodies = Wilson disease

63. This is zinc deficiency. Zinc deficiency is especially common in patients with Crohn's disease and is also seen in alcoholics (beer drinkers, in particular, as beer contains virtually no zinc). In the past, zinc deficiency was also seen in patients on total parenteral nutrition (TPN) therapy, when zinc was not routinely added to the formulation. Zinc may also be sequestered in the liver during episodes of physiological stress, including trauma, infection, and other acute systemic inflammatory conditions. In these instances, there is not a true deficiency but a functional deficiency, as the zinc is maldistributed. The deficiency in Crohn's disease appears to be due to poor zinc absorption, but it may also arise from underlying inflammation with a functional deficiency. Zinc deficiency leads to a characteristic acral-predominant skin lesion that appears as an erythematous, scaling, vesicopustular plaque on the legs and face. It's also associated with diarrhea, as occurred here. The lesions can rapidly improve with appropriate zinc supplementation. ALP is a zinc-metalloenzyme that requires magnesium for activity, so deficiencies of either zinc or magnesium can lead to diminished ALP activity in serum and tissue.

Here's the Point!

Crohn's disease + Low ALP = Zinc deficiency

In addition to the conditions described in Vignettes 60 to 63, diminished ALP has been associated with a number of other clinical conditions and settings. For example, low ALP is commonly observed following cardiac surgery with cardiopulmonary bypass. The mechanism of diminished ALP in this setting is unclear, but it may have something to do with the bypass itself. In addition, it has been reported in vitamin C deficiency (ie, scurvy), in folic acid deficiency, and with low levels of phosphorus. Some patients with celiac sprue have a low ALP (probably from vitamin and micronutrient malabsorption), and it has also been seen in chronic anemia (mechanism also unclear). Table 63-1 provides a full list of conditions that have been associated with diminished ALP levels.

Table 63-1.
CONDITIONS ASSOCIATED WITH LOW ALKALINE PHOSPHATASE LEVELS *(IN NO PARTICULAR ORDER)*
Zinc deficiency
Magnesium deficiency
Vitamin C deficiency/scurvy
Folic acid deficiency
Vitamin B$_6$ deficiency
Excess vitamin D ingestion
Low phosphorus levels, as seen in hypophosphatasia
Celiac disease
Pernicious anemia
Protein-calorie malnutrition
Hypothyroidism
Acute Wilson disease
Cardiac surgery and cardiopulmonary bypass
Severe anemia
Milk-alkali syndrome
Hypoparathyroidism

Vignette 64: Poor Response to Interferon/Ribavirin

A 54-year-old man with genotype 1 hepatitis C virus (HCV) is started on combination therapy with pegylated interferon and ribavirin. The patient is compliant with the medication. HCV RNA is measured at week 12 and remains detectable. There has been a 1-log reduction in HCV RNA from the pretreatment baseline level to the week 12 level.

▶ *How do you classify this response?*
▶ *Should you continue therapy?*

Vignette 64: Answer

This patient has a null response at 12 weeks, and treatment should be discontinued. This vignette provides an excuse to review the frequency for measuring HCV RNA levels during treatment for HCV, and interpretation of the viral kinetics. Early virologic response, or EVR, is defined by a 2-log drop or more in HCV RNA level at week 12. This week 12 milestone has a high predictive value for achieving sustained virologic response (SVR), defined as absent HCV RNA 6 months after treatment cessation. If a patient with genotype 1 HCV achieves EVR, then the SVR rate is around 66%, which is pretty good (Table 64-1). In contrast, if a patient with genotype 1 HCV fails to achieve EVR, then the SVR rate is virtually nil. For this reason, failure to achieve EVR is called a "null response." Patients failing to achieve EVR should not continue therapy. This is one category of not responding to therapy.

The EVR has now been supplemented with another assessment, the rapid virologic response, or RVR. The first benchmark to check following the initiation of HCV treatment, RVR is defined as having an undetectable HCV RNA at week 4 of treatment. If a patient with genotype 1 HCV achieves an RVR at week 4, then the SVR rate approaches a blistering 90%. The same can be said for genotypes 2 and 3. So, if a patient achieves an RVR, he or she should obviously continue the therapy—for a total of 48 weeks for genotype 1 and 24 weeks for genotypes 2 and 3. RVR is achieved in around 25% of patients with genotype 1 and in upwards of 66% of patients with genotypes 2 and 3.

What if patients with genotype 1 achieve an EVR but still have detectable virus by week 24? These patients are also called nonresponders because even though they had a 2-log drop at the 12-week milestone, they did not clear the virus at the critical 24-week milestone. In this circumstance, there is virtually no chance of achieving SVR by week 48, and these patients need to stop therapy. By the way, a "complete EVR" is defined as undetectable virus (not just a 2-log drop) at the 12-week mark and predicts about a 70% SVR after 48 weeks of therapy, which is almost as encouraging as an RVR.

Let's take this one step further. A "partial EVR" is defined as having at least a 2-log drop in virus at 12 weeks but still having detectable HCV RNA until the 24-week mark, where the virus is cleared. These patients, called *slow responders*, have double the relapse compared with the "complete EVR" patients. Therefore, it is now recommended to extend therapy for 72 weeks in these patients. To repeat: if a patient is a slow responder but does finally have negative HCV RNA by week 24, you should extend therapy to 72 weeks instead of the usual 48 weeks for genotype 1 HCV.

Figure 64-1 provides a visual overview of the major patterns of HCV response. Table 64-1 provides more information on how to manage these patients.

Table 64-1.

INTERPRETATION AND TREATMENT APPROACH FOR HCV RNA LEVELS DURING TREATMENT WITH INTERFERON AND RIBAVIRIN*

Week First Became HCV RNA Undetectable	Description	% of Patients	Relapse Rate	SVR Rate	Treatment Strategy
GENOTYPE 1					
4	Rapid response	15	10	90	Keep patients on treatment for 48 weeks even if have to reduce dose. If shorten therapy, SVR still very high
12	Early response	35	33	66	Complete 48 weeks of treatment
24	Slow to respond	15	55	45	Extend therapy to 72 weeks
Never	Null response	20	0	0	Stop treatment as soon as pattern recognized at 12 weeks
Never	Nonresponse	15	0	0	Stop treatment as soon as pattern recognized at 24 weeks
GENOTYPES 2 AND 3					
4	Rapid response	66	10	90	Keep patients on treatment for 24 weeks even if have to reduce dose. If shorten therapy, SVR still very high
After week 4	Early response	33	50	50	Consider extending therapy to 48 weeks
Never	Nonresponse	3	0	0	Stop treatment as soon as pattern recognized at 12 weeks

*Adapted from Schiffman, M. (2008), *Curbside Consultation of the Liver.* Thorofare, NJ: SLACK Incorporated.

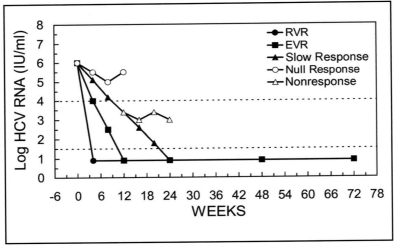

Figure 64-1. Patterns of HCV RNA in patients receiving interferon and riba-virin. (Adapted from Schiffman, M. [2008], *Curbside Consultation of the Liver.* Thorofare, NJ: SLACK Incorporated.)

Why Might This Be Tested? You know that viral hepatitis will be on the exam. These viral kinetics and treatment milestones are perfect for a Board exam because they are tried and true and they set up numerous opportunities for clinical threshold questions. You simply need to memorize this information; every so often the Board exam rewards pure memorization.

Clinical Threshold Alert: EVR requires at least a 2-log drop in HCV RNA versus baseline by week 12 of interferon and ribavirin therapy. Anything less than a 2-log drop by week 12 is a null response. RVR is assessed at 4 weeks. SVR is assessed 6 months after cessation of treatment. Genotype 1 slow responders should receive 72 weeks of therapy, not 48 weeks.

Here's the Point!

If a patient with genotype 1 HCV does not achieve EVR, stop therapy. Also, just know Table 64-1!

Here's the Point!

Genotype 1 slow responders should be treated for 72 weeks.

Vignette 65: Oral Contraceptives and a Liver Mass

A 32-year-old woman presents to her primary care provider with dyspepsia. Her initial workup includes an abdominal ultrasound, which reveals a 7 x 6 cm mass at the edge of the liver. A follow-up MRI confirms the lesion and demonstrates that it's situated beneath the liver capsule (Figure 65-1). The mass lights up on the arterial phase of imaging and is otherwise homogeneous. There is no evidence of cirrhosis on imaging, physical examination, or biochemical testing. AFP level is normal. The patient has been taking an oral contraceptive for 5 years.

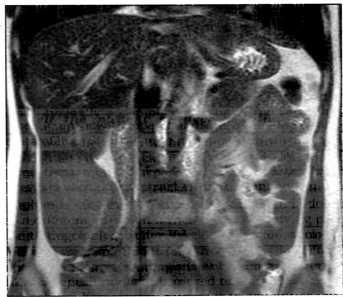

Figure 65-1. Subcapsular liver lesion drooping off the right lobe of the liver.

▶ *How should you manage this lesion?*

Vignette 65: Answer

This is a hepatic adenoma. You probably knew that. The key features of hepatic adenoma include the exposure to oral contraceptives and the enhancement on arterial phase of MRI. In addition, hepatic adenomas are frequently (but not universally) subcapsular in location. The lack of a central scar argues against something like focal nodular hyperplasia or fibrolamellar hepatocellular cancer (see Vignette 25 for more on those lesions).

The question asked, however, is how you should manage the lesion, which is a little more tricky. Hepatic adenomas are benign, but because they are often subcapsular and highly vascular, they can spontaneously rupture. When they rupture, they can lead to massive exsanguination into the peritoneal cavity. The risk of hemorrhage increases to about 30% as the adenoma enlarges, and the bleeding itself has a 6% mortality rate. In addition, hepatic adenomas can transform into cancer. For these reasons, surgical resection is the treatment of choice when feasible.

Hepatic adenomas are strongly associated with oral contraception use (as mentioned earlier) and also anabolic steroid use (as is peliosis hepatis—see Vignette 20), so the offending agent must be discontinued when this type of lesion is identified. In fact, these lesions were exceedingly rare before the advent of the birth control pill and anabloic steroids. Although hepatic adenomas can regress after discontinuation of oral contraceptives, there are reports of rare malignant transformation in some hepatic adenomas that regress. Thus, if they are reachable, they should be resected. However, some adenomas can be in difficult spots, like the porta hepatis. In such cases, it may be reasonable to follow the smaller adenomas (ie, <5 cm) after oral contraceptives have been discontinued. Because that is controversial, it's unlikely to be the subject of an exam question. But you certainly should know the diagnosis and its association with oral contraceptives. And for larger lesions (≥5 cm), there is little debate that surgical resection is warranted even if oral contraceptives are discontinued.

So for the patient in the current vignette, there are 2 good reasons to remove the lesion. First, it's symptomatic and, second, it's large; discontinuing the oral contraceptive is not enough. It's important to advise patients with hepatic adenomas to avoid becoming pregnant. These adenomas can grow during pregnancy with the risk of massive hemorrhage. For that reason, all adenomas should be resected prior to a planned pregnancy.

Why Might This Be Tested? Liver masses, in general, are nearly guaranteed to be on the Board exam. So we've included a variety of liver masses throughout this book. In addition, you can find several other vignettes pertaining to liver masses in the original *Acing the GI Board Exam* book. The hepatic adenoma is a classic. The trick here is to not just accurately identify this fairly obvious diagnosis, but to figure what to do with it; the latter is what we call a "second-level" question that goes beyond the mere diagnosis.

Here's the Point!

Oral contraceptive + Subcapsular liver mass = Hepatic adenoma

Vignette 66: Can't Lose Weight

A 35-year-old man is referred to you for management of elevated aminotransferases in the setting of diabetes and hyperlipidemia. He began treatment for diabetes 8 years ago and is now insulin dependent. He first developed elevated aminotransferases 5 years ago, at which time his BMI was 41. He attempted to lose weight on several occasions, including under a supervised program, but his current BMI is 42. He is adamant that he "can't lose weight" despite focused attempts at weight loss. His only medications are simvastatin and insulin. He does not drink alcohol. His most recent liver tests include the following values: AST = 96, ALT = 125, ALP = 63, total bilirubin = 1.3, and INR = 1.0. You now obtain a liver biopsy, which is pictured in Figure 66-1.

Figure 66-1. Liver biopsy for patient in Vignette 66. (Reprinted with permission of Alton B. Farris, MD, Emory University.)

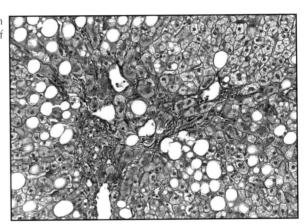

▶ *How should this be managed?*

Vignette 66: Answer

This is nonalcoholic fatty liver disease, or NAFLD. We provided an overview of NAFLD in Vignette 37, including the grades of steatohepatitis. Remember that NAFLD is part of the metabolic syndrome, a condition marked by insulin resistance with hyperglycemia, hyperlipidemia, hypertension, and atherosclerotic cardiovascular disease. The metabolic syndrome is usually diagnosed clinically on the basis of these comorbidities, and NAFLD runs with the pack. But metabolic syndrome can also be diagnosed more formally by measuring insulin resistance using the homeostatic model assessment (HOMA), which is a mathematical model that yields a score based on fasting plasma glucose and insulin concentrations. The details of HOMA are beyond the scope of this mini-review, but suffice it to say that HOMA works well as an inexpensive and easily calculated alternative to the more laborious euglycemic glucose clamp method of estimating insulin resistance.

Whether diagnosed clinically, by HOMA, or by both means, insulin resistance causes big-time trouble. NAFLD is one of the various complications of insulin resistance. Although NAFLD may occur in nonobese patients, it's overwhelmingly found in obese patients with metabolic syndrome.

Recall that NAFLD is defined as hepatic steatosis (with or without steatohepatitis) exceeding 5% to 10% of the liver mass in the absence of significant alcohol consumption. The patient in this vignette has more than NAFLD—he has NASH. His liver biopsy with trichrome stain, depicted in Figure 66-1, reveals steatosis, lobular inflammation, ballooning hepatocytes (steatohepatitis) within a mesh of "chicken-wire" fibrosis. Cirrhosis may be right around the corner if this continues.

This scenario is incredibly common. The Framingham heart study revealed that around 50% of the American populace is now overweight, and 1 in 4 Americans is obese. Obesity is an overwhelming public health issue, and gastroenterologists and hepatologists are on the front lines of this epidemic. You can bet that the Board exam will include questions about the management of obesity, especially in patients with advancing liver disease. You might not have signed up to become a dietitian or endocrinologist, but—like it or not—that is now part of your identity.

The good news is that weight loss may abate the progression of NASH to cirrhosis in this patient. But despite supervised attempts at weight loss, he has not been able to shed the pounds. He has a BMI of 42, which is class III obesity—otherwise known as severe, extreme, or morbid obesity. Table 66-1 provides the full classification for BMI as supported by the National Institutes of Health (NIH) and the World Health Organization. It's amazing how many people consider a BMI of 30 to be "normal." As shown in the table, a BMI of 30 is actually class I obesity. A normal BMI is between 18.5 and 24.9.

Table 66-1. BODY MASS INDEX CLASSIFICATIONS ADOPTED BY THE NATIONAL INSTITUTES OF HEALTH AND THE WORLD HEALTH ORGANIZATION	
BMI Range	Classification
<18.5 kg/m^2	Underweight
>18.5 to 24.9 kg/m^2	Normal
>25 to 29.9 kg/m^2	Overweight
>30 to 34.9 kg/m^2	Obesity Class I
>35 to 39.9 kg/m^2	Obesity Class II
>40 kg/m^2	Obesity Class III (extreme, severe, or morbid obesity)

The BMI is preferred over body weight as a measure of obesity because it better correlates with the percentage of body fat, in particular. Plus, the BMI is much more predictive of obesity complications, including mortality, than weight alone. One caveat about the BMI is that it's less accurate in patients who are big yet muscular—these bodybuilder types have much less body fat than the BMI would predict. For the rest of us, though, the BMI works pretty well as a quick estimate of body fat mass. Another caveat is that the thresholds in Table 66-1 were developed from data on Caucasians. Different races should probably have different cutoffs. For example, in people of South Asian decent, the risks of obesity begin to mount at much lower BMI cutoffs than in Caucasians. This partly explains why NAFLD is more common in nonobese Asians compared to nonobese individuals of other races. In contrast, obesity-related complications accumulate at higher BMI thresholds in African-Americans than in Caucasians.

While we are on the topic of obesity assessment, it's important to note that the BMI is only part of the evaluation process. The United States Preventive Services Task Force (USPSTF) and The National Institues of Health (NIH), among others, suggest measuring waist circumference in addition to BMI. The idea behind waist circumference is that it estimates abdominal fat, in particular—and central adiposity (also called "android" adiposity) is classically associated with an increased risk of diabetes, high blood pressure, cardiovascular disease, and hyperlipidemia. In patients who are overweight or have class I obesity, the risk of obesity complications rise when the waist circumference exceeds 40 inches in men and 35 inches in women. These are good numbers to keep in mind for clinical practice, although we doubt they will be directly tested on the GI Board exam. But certainly know that waist circumference correlates with central adiposity, which, in turn, is highly related to cardiovascular complications of obesity. Once patients reach class II obesity or beyond (eg, BMI >35), the waist circumference does not provide much additional explanatory power; at that point the BMI alone tells the story.

So, this patient is morbidly obese, and he has remained morbidly obese despite supervised attempts at weight loss. He is young and has evidence of advanced complications of obesity, including NASH. This vignette asked how this patient should be managed. Given his age, failure to lose weight, and mounting complications, you should recommend bariatric surgery. Medical therapy (which is still evolving) and diets just won't cut it. If he doesn't lose weight, he will likely die much sooner than he otherwise should. This is a tragedy waiting to happen, so you must be prepared to discuss bariatric surgery and refer him to the appropriate consultants. This vignette underscores the utility of a liver biopsy. Despite the risks associated with liver biopsy, such as bleeding, the diagnostic value supersedes the risk in this situation. Just checking this patient's liver tests annually would not help.

Bariatric surgery is effective. Although there are a variety of possible complications, bariatric surgery is the most effective approach for managing morbid obesity. In patients who are morbidly obese, surgery improves survival and enhances overall quality of life. Bariatric surgery is indicated for patients with a BMI >40 or a BMI $\geq$35 with comorbid complications. Importantly, bariatric surgery has recently been shown to improve steatosis, necroinflammation, and even hepatic fibrosis in NASH. Although every patient does not experience these results, most exhibit improvements in histologic parameters as long as the weight loss is not too rapid.

Not all bariatric surgeries are created equal. In the past, surgeons would fashion a jejunoileal bypass in which the intestinal anastomosis was placed just proximal to the ileocecal valve. This was highly effective for weight loss, as you can imagine, but was rife with complications. In particular, many patients developed liver failure following the operation, so the jejunoileal bypass is now long gone.

Laparoscopic adjustable gastric banding (LAGB) has become very popular because of its relative ease of placement and low risk of complications. In the LAGB operation, a circumferential band is placed around the stomach to create a restrictive pouch. This works pretty well for weight loss but is not as effective for reversing the metabolic complications of obesity compared to other operations. This is likely attributed to the fact that LAGB does not change hormonal profiles the way other approaches can.

The Roux-en-Y gastric bypass (RYGB), which is now the operation of choice for morbidly obese patients and those with advanced metabolic complications of obesity, provides robust weight loss *and* improvements in metabolic parameters. In the RYGB, a 15- to 20-mL restrictive pouch is created in the stomach, and the Roux loop is brought up to the pouch. As a result, the duodenum and proximal jejunum are bypassed. This duodenal bypass may be the magic ingredient for reducing metabolic complications, possibly because duodenal passage of gastric contents triggers a cascade of regulatory peptides. The LAGB, in contrast, does not alter the hormonal milieu in the same manner, since duodenal transit is retained.

In any event, this young man needs surgery. Without it he could die young, but with an effective operation coupled with postoperative counseling and oversight, he might reverse the NAFLD, cure his diabetes, improve his quality of life, and even prolong his life span.

Why Might This Be Tested? You can expect to see this on the exam. You should know all about NAFLD as the hepatic manifestation of metabolic syndrome, and you should know all about the obesity epidemic.

Clinical Threshold Alert: A BMI between 25 and 29.9 is "overweight." A BMI above 30 is "obese."

Here's the Point!

Bariatric surgery is the most effective therapy for a morbidly obese patient with NASH who is unable to lose weight via traditional methods.

Vignette 67: Pregnancy Consultation

A 28-year-old primigravid woman at 30 weeks' gestation presents to you for further evaluation. She has been feeling particularly fatigued over the past 2 weeks and has noticed skin changes. She also has mild nausea but has been eating small amounts without vomiting. She complains of polyuria. She had terrible nocturnal heartburn earlier in this pregnancy and had been under the care of another gastroenterologist (until she appeared at your office today). In review of those records, you find that an upper endoscopy was performed in the second trimester that showed small esophageal varices without red signs, a sliding hiatal hernia, and no evidence of erosive esophagitis. Recent laboratory workup for liver disease was unremarkable, and there is no family or personal history of liver disease. Her retrosternal pyrosis has resolved with the use of a proton pump inhibitor daily. There has been no hematochezia, melena, diarrhea, hematemesis, or weight loss. She has not had fevers, rigors, pruritus, or jaundice.

She saw her primary care physician yesterday, and laboratory tests were ordered. She was referred to see you the very next day.

Her vital signs show a temperature of 98.8°F, blood pressure of 92/60, heart rate of 100, and respiratory rate of 18. Physical examination reveals bilateral palmar erythema, a few spider angiomas, a gravid abdomen, trace pitting edema, and varicosities of the lower extremities. No other remarkable findings are noted on examination. Laboratory tests reveal the following: albumin = 3.3, total bilirubin = 1.0, ALT = 21, AST = 18, GGT = 22, ALP = 290, BUN = 5, creatinine = 0.5, glucose = 80, WBC = 4.9, hemoglobin = 11.2, MCV = 92, platelets = 190, normal serum bile acids, and normal urinalysis. Doppler ultrasound of the abdomen reveals a normal-appearing liver, spleen, and vasculature without ascites.

▶ **What is the diagnosis?**

▶ **What needs to be done now?**

Vignette 67: Answer

I know what you're thinking: pregnancy, pregnancy, pregnancy. You might as well be preparing for the obstetrics Board examination. As we've said before, pregnancy seems to come up over and over on the GI Board exam. Remember that most adult women get pregnant and have the potential to face some liver issues during this time. Obstetricians will refer these challenges to gastroenterologists (and rightly so). So pregnancy presents dilemmas that commonly face the GI practitioner. Quite simply, you need to know this stuff cold.

So, back to the vignette. Don't be fooled here; this is a *normal* pregnancy. The patient should be followed expectantly by her obstetrician, and no further tests are needed at this time. A certain level of paranoia is understandable since you are dealing with two lives: mother and fetus. However, this case demonstrates typical and expected findings with normal pregnancy. The physiologic changes that occur with pregnancy are important to understand, and are worth reviewing here, since you need to be able to recognize them when bad things really do happen.

Let's break this case down further. This patient's fatigue is most likely from the increased energy demands of pregnancy. Although nausea is nonspecific and can have many causes, here it's most likely due to gastric compression from an enlarging uterus. The patient is compensating by eating smaller amounts. Polyuria is probably from urinary bladder compression, also from the enlarging uterus. Furthermore, the uterine enlargement interferes with venous return from the lower extremities and is leading to her edema and varicose veins. There is up to a 50% increase in cardiac output in pregnancy, mostly due to increased plasma volume, which raises the heart rate as the gestation advances. This increase in plasma volume causes hemodilution and results in the relatively low albumin, hemoglobin, BUN, and creatinine levels. The slightly low blood pressure is due to systemic vasodilation; however, the blood pressure tends to gradually increase further along in the gestation. Palmar erythema and spider angiomas are commonly found during pregnancy due to the increased estrogen levels. The elevation of the ALP results from the addition of placental ALP (notice that the GGT level was normal). The presence of small esophageal varices can be found in up to half of healthy pregnant patients due to increased flow in the veins of the azygos system (which feed esophagogastric varices). However, these varices do not typically bleed. We could have also thrown in an elevated AFP level (which is also normal in pregnancy), but we thought we had confused you enough already. Therefore, you have a normal pregnant patient here and you can advise her primary care provider to relax and not worry at this point in time.

Why Might This Be Tested? You have to know the basic physiologic changes of pregnancy to understand when there is real pathology. There is no need to be intimidated when you see a question about a pregnant patient or when you get a consult on a gravid patient in real life. If you know your stuff, you will be more confident and able to answer the query right away. Remember, confidence breeds success (so long as it's not false confidence)!

Here's the Point!

Elevated ALP in pregnancy is due to the addition of placental ALP.

Here's the Point!

Palmar erythema and spider angiomas can be seen in normal pregnancy due to the elevated serum estrogen levels.

Here's the Point!

Small esophageal varices can form during pregnancy due to increased flow in the azygos system—these do not typically bleed.

Vignette 68: The Itchy and Scratchy Show

A 38-year-old man is referred to you for further evaluation of abnormal liver tests. Review of systems reveals flushing with alcohol ingestion, intermittent abdominal pain, and bouts of diarrhea. Upon further questioning, you learn that he can literally write on his skin during periods of flushing, leaving visible red streaks where he scratches with his fingernails. Physical exam is notable for hepatosplenomegaly. Labs reveal an elevated ALP and GGT.

▸ *What is the most likely diagnosis?*

Vignette 68: Answer

This is systemic mastocytosis. This condition is a Board favorite because it presents in many different ways and affects nearly every major organ system. Although mastocytosis often infiltrates the liver, it's a systemic disorder characterized by mast cell infiltration of several systems including lymph nodes, spleen, skin, bone marrow, central nervous system, and the GI tract. The high ALP occurs because of diffuse infiltration of the liver with mast cells. Recall that anything that diffusely infiltrates the liver can drive up the ALP, often out of proportion to the aminotransferases. The mast cell infiltrates secrete histamine, which, in turn, can lead to hypersecretion of acid in the stomach, peptic ulcers, and acid reflux disease. This is a rare hyperacidic syndrome that can be treated as effectively with a histamine-2 receptor blocker as with a proton pump inhibitor. Mastocytosis can lead to periodic flushing (particularly with alcohol ingestion), abdominal pain, diarrhea with malabsorption, paresthesias, low blood pressure (histamine mediated), and just about anything else! A fun fact is that it's associated with Darier's sign, which is visible urticaria from scratching the skin (ie, dermatographism). By the way, if you don't recognize the source of this vignette's title, it's time to bone up on your Simpson's trivia.

Why Might This Be Tested? Because it's extremely rare, and the Board examiners seem to love testing rare diagnoses; knowledge of rare diagnoses extracts the true "acers" from the rest of the crowd. Plus Board examiners seem to love questions on dermatologic manifestations of GI disorders.

Here's the Point!

Big liver + Flushing + Dermatographism + High ALP = Mastocytosis

Vignette 69: D-Penicillamine Trouble

A patient with recently diagnosed Wilson disease is started on D-penicillamine therapy to manage serum copper levels. The patient develops a fever and cutaneous skin eruptions within days. He presents for evaluation and is found to have new lymphadenopathy on physical exam. Laboratories reveal new thrombocytopenia and neutropenia.

▶ **What happened here?**
▶ **How should this patient be managed, both acutely and chronically?**

Vignette 69: Answer

This is an early hypersensitivity reaction to D-penicillamine, which is known to occur in up to 10% of patients started on this therapy. D-penicillamine is an orally administered chelating agent that helps reduce copper levels by promoting copper excretion in the urine. It's an amazing drug because it can reverse neurologic symptoms in Wilson disease, slow overall disease progression, and significantly extend overall survival. But these remarkable benefits come with a price; there are many serious side effects of D-penicillamine (which is the main reason that another chelator with fewer side effects, trientine, has gained favor). The adverse events of D-penicillamine are traditionally divided into early versus late-occurring consequences. The current vignette demonstrates the most serious early adverse event, which is a hypersensitivity reaction marked by fever, skin rash, lymphadenopathy, thrombocytopenia, and neutropenia. This reaction usually occurs within 3 weeks of starting therapy. When hypersensitivity occurs, the drug must be stopped immediately. Some advocate restarting the therapy with the addition of steroids, but that is a matter of personal style, the severity of the initial reaction, and knowing the patient. Late adverse events are multiple and include Goodpasture's syndrome, pemphigoid lesions, lichen planus, and a lupus-like syndrome, among others. Also keep in mind (as noted in Vignette 36) that both neurologic symptoms and liver tests may initially worsen after starting D-penicillamine, but subsequent improvement typically occurs within 6 months of starting therapy (ie, it takes a while for it to work, so don't stop the medicine if the symptoms initially worsen unless there is a serious side effect like a hypersensitivity reaction).

Since this patient did not tolerate D-penicillamine, the next step is to use an alternative chelating agent or zinc salts (or both). Trientine is less potent than D-penicillamine but has a much more favorable side-effect profile, and in many patients trientine is as effective as D-penicillamine. Zinc salts have a different mechanism of action than the chelators. Rather than binding up copper, zinc blocks intestinal absorption of copper and basically traps the copper within the enterocytes. Also keep in mind that patients with Wilson disease should avoid copper-rich foods (as discussed in Vignette 12), such as those listed in Table 69-1.

Why Might This Be Tested? The emphasis of a disease on the Board exam often seems to be inversely proportional to its population prevalence. Since Wilson disease is very rare, you had better know it well! There are just too many nuances and pearls to think that Wilson disease will not be on the exam.

Table 69-1. COPPER-RICH FOODS TO AVOID IN WILSON DISEASE (IN NO PARTICULAR ORDER)	
Chocolate	Navy beans
Sesame seeds	Garbanzo beans
Raw cashews	Soybeans
Sunflower seeds	Cooked barley
Poppy seeds	Oysters
Liver (go figure!)	

Here's the Point!

D-penicillamine causes many side effects. Most patients can be treated with trientine and/or zinc salts.

Vignettes 70 to 75: Cirrhosis/Renal Throw Down

It's hard to find a patient with decompensated cirrhosis who does not have, or is not soon to have, some kidney trouble. It can be vexing to sort out what's causing elevated creatinine levels and azotemia in these patients. The differential diagnosis is extensive; it includes not only the usual causes of renal failure, but also the cirrhosis-specific etiologies. This can get confusing, so what better topic to put on a Board exam? Let's just mix it up and jump in. This renal throw down will help you see where you are with your renal knowledge *vis-à-vis* cirrhosis. In each mini-vignette in the following series, identify the most likely cause of the elevated creatinine.

70. A 72-year-old patient with cirrhosis and a MELD score of 13 complicated by diuretic-controlled ascites is found to have grade 1 hepatic encephalopathy at a clinic visit. The patient normally receives furosemide 80 mg daily and spironolactone 200 mg daily for control of ascites, which has been effective. Baseline creatinine is 1.0. Sodium and potassium balance has been well preserved. At the clinic visit, the serum bicarbonate is 27 mEq/L. A spot urine revealed a sodium: potassium ratio exceeding 1.0 and a spot urine sodium of 20 mmol/L. The patient is started on oral neomycin, which helps the encephalopathy. However, on follow-up lab testing, the creatinine has risen to 2.3. There has been no interval change in diuretic dosing. What happened here? And what else do you need to screen for to cover the bases? (This is a "read our mind" or "Do you hear us?" type of question, but think about it for a second...)

71. A patient with tense ascites undergoes paracentesis that yields 18 L of fluid. She is then started on strict sodium restriction and diuretic therapy, beginning with furosemide 40 mg daily and spironolactone 100 mg daily. The ascites does not improve, and a spot urine sodium is 5 mmol/L, with a urine sodium:potassium ratio below 1.0. The diuretics are increased, and she is concurrently treated with serial large-volume paracenteses. But these measures do not help—the ascites persists. The diuretic dose is gradually pushed to 160 mg daily of furosemide and 400 mg daily of spironolactone. At this level, the creatinine rises from a baseline of 1.0 to its current level of 2.3. The fractional excretion of sodium (FENa) is low, and the bicarbonate is elevated at 32. The patient is also noted to be increasingly encephalopathic in parallel with the increase in diuretic dosage. What is the most likely reason for the elevated creatinine, and what is the next step in managing this patient?

72. A patient with well-compensated cirrhosis and a MELD score of 7 has a normal baseline creatinine of 1.0. He injures his ankle and reports to the emergency department (ED) for evaluation, where he is ruled out for a fracture and is placed on a course of therapy to help manage a severely sprained ankle. A week later he undergoes routine lab testing by his primary care provider. His creatinine is now 2.3. What is your best guess about what happened here? Imagine that you are on the phone right now with the primary care provider, who has "curbsided" you.

73. A 61-year-old with well-compensated cirrhosis from chronic hepatitis C develops new-onset ankle edema. He presents to his primary care physician, who orders labs that reveal the following: creatinine = 2.3 (baseline = 1.0); albumin = 1.8 (baseline = 3.1), AST = 48, ALT = 53, total bilirubin = 1.6, INR = 1.3. The patient is referred to his gastroenterologist, who checks a 24-hour urine protein (4.6 g), serum complement levels (low), and a rheumatoid factor (positive). What is the most likely explanation for this picture?

74. A patient with cirrhosis and ascites develops low-grade fevers and abdominal pain. Paracentesis is performed and reveals a total PMN count of 550. Cultures grow out *Escherichia coli*. Laboratories are checked, which reveal a creatinine of 2.3 (baseline = 1.0). What might be causing the acute renal insufficiency here?

75. The patient in Vignette 71 starts to require weekly paracentesis with intravenous albumin. The diuretics are discontinued to avoid further contraction alkalosis. However, the creatinine begins to rise further. Within 2 weeks, the creatinine has risen to 3.2, and the creatinine clearance is estimated to be 10 mL/min. The urine output begins to drop, culminating in oliguria. The urine sediment is bland without evidence of casts or erythrocytes. There are no other obvious nephrotoxins on board. The patient does not have evidence of spontaneous bacterial peritonitis, other infections, GI bleeding, or shock. What is the most likely diagnosis? How should this be treated?

Vignettes 70 to 75: Answers

70. This is neomycin-induced renal toxicity. Although neomycin historically has been used for managing the symptoms of hepatic encephalopathy, it's not commonly used anymore given the availability of safer alternatives (see Vignette 11 for more details). Neomycin can cause renal toxicity; it even has a black box warning from the FDA regarding this adverse event. Several risk factors raise the likelihood of developing renal failure from neomycin. These include advanced age (as seen here), pre-existing renal impairment (not seen here), and use of diuretic therapy and/or volume depletion (seen here). This patient is on a reasonably high dose of diuretic therapy, and although it has been effective, there is evidence of some contraction alkalosis (bicarb slightly elevated). This patient seemed okay on the regimen before the neomycin was given; that is, the patient was otherwise stable, the ascites was controlled, and the creatinine was normal. Also, there was adequate urine sodium excretion, based on the urine indices (see the other mini-vignettes in this series for more on interpreting the urine indices). But this patient became a perfect setup for kidney trouble due to his age, underlying cirrhosis (which itself is a setup for renal injury, as discussed further below), and diuresis. Neomycin probably should not have been used here. As for what else you should screen for, the answer is that you need to screen for ototoxicity by asking about hearing and tinnitus symptoms. Although nephrotoxicity and ototoxicity do not go hand in hand, you need to screen for ototoxicity nonetheless.

Here's the Point!

Predictors of neomycin-induced kidney injury in cirrhosis:
- Advanced age
- Preexisting renal insufficiency
- Volume depletion
- Use of diuretics

71. This is contraction alkalosis and renal insufficiency resulting from over-diuresis. This patient has diuretic-resistant, refractory ascites defined as persistent ascites despite sodium restriction and maximal doses of oral diuretics. It has been nearly 50 years since investigators determined that the maximum physiologic rate of peritoneal fluid absorption is 500 mL per day. That is an important number to keep in mind because it indicates a physiologic ceiling for how fast ascitic fluid can be mobilized. When there is a lot of extravascular volume marked by peripheral edema, diuretics work fine to keep the fluid moving along. But once that fluid is mobilized, the ascites becomes the main focus. So it then becomes a race to see if the fluid removal from the peritoneum (physiologically capped at about 500 mL per day) can outpace the rate of fluid collection in the peritoneum. As cirrhosis gets worse and worse, portal hypertension and systemic arterial vasodilation increase in tandem. This leads to renal hypoperfusion with compensatory sodium and free water retention by the kidney. So the race begins as the body absorbs more and more sodium and water, and the diuretics try to dump the sodium and water out. In the meantime the ascites just keeps on accumulating, and at some point the rate of accumulation exceeds the physiologic ceiling of reabsorption. So what happens then? Well, if you keep flogging with diuretics, it will just serve to totally dry out the patient. Since the ascitic fluid just can't be sucked out any faster than 500 mL per day, other fluid spaces get drained instead (namely diuresis from the intravascular space coupled with the increasing systemic vasoconstriction). And then the patient experiences even more intravascular volume depletion, develops a contraction alkalosis, and bumps the creatinine as a consequence of prerenal azotemia. This is marked by a low FENa and low urine sodium (below 10 mmol/L). Patients may also develop worsening hepatic encephalopathy in the setting of contraction alkalosis, as occurred here.

So the treatment is not to push the diuretics any further. Instead, you should stop the diuretics, acknowledge pharmacologic defeat, and replete the intravascular volume with intravenous albumin or other colloid. As far as treatment for the ascites is concerned, serial large-volume paracentesis or TIPS can be considered. Ultimately liver transplantation is the only treatment that can improve survival when this chain of events begins to unfold.

Here's the Point!

Understand Figure 71-1, below.

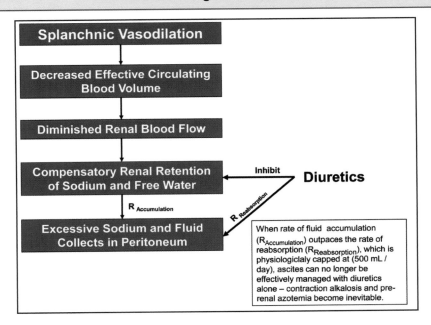

72. It is hard to know for sure what happened here because the vignette does not provide quite enough information. But if you think about it, the ED probably started this patient on a NSAID to manage the sprained ankle. Under normal circumstances, it's not a big deal to begin a NSAID in someone with an ankle sprain. But in a patient with cirrhosis you always need to think about what medicines you are giving and what the consequences might be. The neomycin example in Vignette 70 is a classic; this is another. NSAIDs can cause acute kidney injury even in healthy individuals, but patients with cirrhosis are especially prone to acute kidney injury even if they are otherwise well. That does not mean that NSAIDs can never be used in a patient with cirrhosis (although you better be watching very closely if such a patient is on an NSAID); but the NSAID should definitely be stopped if there is a bump in the creatinine.

73. This is mixed cryoglobulinemia from hepatitis C. See Vignette 24 for more information about cryoglobulinemia. Clues here include the low complement levels, proteinuria, and positive rheumatoid factor. Other clues that are not seen here include a purpuric rash from leukocytoclastic vasculitis, paresthesias from peripheral neuropathy, and abdominal pain from vasculitis. The renal involvement in cryoglobulinemia is variable. Here the patient exhibits a nephrotic syndrome, but patients can also present with acute nephritic syndrome, membranoproliferative glomerulonephritis, chronic kidney disease without an obvious glomerulonephropathy, or even acute renal failure. A GI Board exam is unlikely to ask you about the details of the renal injury. Just be aware that it can vary.

Here's the Point!

Hepatitis C + Positive rheumatoid factor + Low complement + Lower extremity purpuric rash + Paresthesias + Renal disease = Mixed cryoglobulinemia

74. This is renal insufficiency from spontaneous bacterial peritonitis (SBP). How can SBP have anything to do with the kidneys? Well, as these vignettes all point out, the kidneys are especially susceptible in cirrhosis. Patients with cirrhosis already have some underlying splanchnic vasodilation, so the kidneys are already a little underperfused. They can handle this if there are no perturbations and life stays the same. But the kidneys can be quickly boxed in if anything disrupts the delicate vascular balance. Infections like SBP can do just that. In SBP there is an accumulation of endotoxins from the smoldering infection, and these can further exaggerate systemic vasodilation. Just a little bit of extra vasodilation might be enough to tip the balance and greatly diminish effective renal perfusion. So, think about a new-onset infection as one of the possible culprits (in addition to everything else that might happen, such as GI bleeding leading to systemic hypotension) whenever the creatinine goes up in a patient with cirrhosis. Along the same lines, ongoing GI bleeding can precipitate hypotension and lead to creatinine elevations as well, so it's important to think about all the different things that can box in the kidneys.

Here's the Point!

Think about a new infection (like SBP) when the creatinine bumps in a patient with cirrhosis (in addition to everything else that causes this!).

75. This is hepatorenal syndrome, or HRS. We could fill the next 30 pages writing about HRS, but we won't. Let's just cover the basics for now. HRS is basically the end result of the cascade depicted in Figure 71-1. To review, as cirrhosis gets worse and worse, systemic vasodilation becomes more prominent (a result of different circulating vasodilators, like nitric oxide, in particular). The effective circulating blood volume drops, there is less blood flow to the kidneys, and renal function declines. The kidneys respond by aggressively retaining sodium and, secondarily, free water. This helps to fill the intravascular space a bit, but not for long; the fluid just starts spilling into extravascular spaces, including the soft tissues (edema) and peritoneum (ascites). Renal function drops even more, the kidneys become even more desperate, and sodium and water reabsorption continue at full throttle. The vicious cycle continues. Finally, the kidneys can't keep up anymore and just give out. But it gets worse. As systemic pressures drop, the body starts to route blood to where it really matters—the brain and heart. Hypotension triggers the renin-angiotensin system and the sympathetic nervous system, and this leads to compensatory vasoconstriction in different vascular beds, including the femoral and renal arteries. That is bad news for the kidneys, not only because they are seeing less perfusion and suffering as a consequence, but also because the afferent arterioles are clamping down at just the wrong moment. The kidneys go from being boxed in to being strangulated by intense afferent vasoconstriction. Now the kidneys maximize sodium and free water absorption, urine sodium levels fall below 10 mEq per day, and the patient develops oliguria (as seen here). Administering a vasopressin analog, like terlipressin (not yet available in the United States), can partly correct the perturbed vascular system by serving to increase the mean arterial pressure, drop renin levels, and improve renal perfusion and glomerular filtration. The net result is to loosen the vice on the kidney, which is evidenced by increased urine sodium concentrations. Combination therapy with midodrine (a selective alpha-1 adrenergic agonist) and octreotide (a somatostatin analog) can also serve this role. Midodrine can work to increase vascular tone and pressures, and octreotide reduces concentrations of splanchnic vasodilators. Further, infusions of albumin can help to increase the effective circulating volume. Basically, however, this is an "all hands on deck" situation, and while these therapies may temporize the situation, only liver transplant will dictate survival.

To make things more complicated, HRS is divided into type I and type II. Just remember that type I is the serious type, and type II is the less serious (but still not great) type and is commonly seen in refractory ascites. In type I HRS things happen fast—there is a ≥50% drop in creatinine clearance to a value below 20 mL/min in a ≤2 week period, or there is a 2-times increase in serum creatinine levels, with a level exceeding 2.5 mg/dL (lots of numbers here—just remember that it happens fast and furious). Type II HRS is a slow-growing phenomenon and is basically the situation in Figure 71-1 before things go haywire; it's having refractory ascites and seeing the creatinine rise in the process. So, type II HRS is similar to the patient described in Vignette 71, although some argue that diuretics cannot precipitate HRS. We won't delve into that physiologic debate here, but will simply say that type II HRS is the end result of refractory ascites, whereas type I involves a rapid decompensation. In both types of HRS you need to rule out other obvious causes of intrinsic renal failure (ie, you need to determine that there is no evidence of glomerulonephritis in urinalysis, no obvious nephrotoxins, no post-renal obstructions, no infections like SBP, no bleeding or shock, etc). That is, HRS is a diagnosis of exclusion. The kidneys in HRS are actually fine—the problem is the prerenal state coupled with the afferent vasoconstriction. Remember that patients with type I HRS are going downhill fast and will receive higher prioritization for liver transplantation (the MELD score rises with the increasing creatinine). Furthermore, they usually do not require a combined liver and kidney transplantation since the kidneys should return to normal function after the liver transplant.

Here's the Point!

Type I HRS = Fast and furious renal decompensation (see text for details)
Type II HRS = Basically refractory ascites with a rising creatinine

(In both cases there is no evidence of intrinsic kidney disease, no obvious nephrotoxins, and no shock, bleeding, or infection.)

Vignette 76: Lots and Lots of Stones

A 48-year-old man who recently immigrated from Mexico is referred for evaluation of jaundice and abnormal liver tests, including the following: ALP = 802, ALT = 135, AST = 141, albumin = 3.4, total bilirubin = 12.8, creatinine = 1.5, INR = 1.1, WBC = 7.3, platelets = 202. Beside noting jaundice, he has been asymptomatic. On examination, he is found to be afebrile with otherwise unremarkable vital signs. The liver and spleen are not palpable, and there is no shifting dullness on abdominal exam. He is icteric, but otherwise there are no stigmata of chronic liver disease and no peripheral edema. Abdominal CT reveals intrahepatic biliary dilatation with multiple intrahepatic stones (Figure 76-1). A follow-up ERCP reveals innumerable stones in the common bile duct and intrahepatic ducts without cholelithiasis (Figure 76-2).

Figure 76-1. Multiple round lucencies in the liver consistent with intrahepatic stones. (Reprinted with permission of Francisco Durazo, MD, Ronald Reagan UCLA Medical Center.)

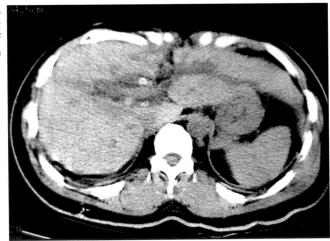

Figure 76-2. ERCP with cholangiogram revealing innumerable space-filling objects in the common bile duct and intrahepatic ducts. (Reprinted with permission of Francisco Durazo, MD, Ronald Reagan UCLA Medical Center.)

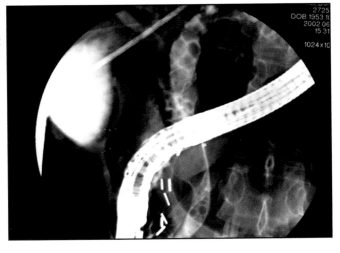

▶ **What is the most likely diagnosis?**

Vignette 76: Answer

This is recurrent pyogenic cholangitis, also known as Oriental cholangitis. For a full review of this condition, refer to the original *Acing* book. In short, pyogenic cholangitis is most commonly seen in Southeast Asians, with a particularly high prevalence in rural areas of China and Hong Kong. However, it also has been diagnosed in Latino immigrants to the United States (as in this case), so its association with Asia is not exclusive (one more reason why the term *Oriental cholangitis* is unfortunate).

The cause of this unusual condition remains unknown. It has been variably blamed on bacterial infections, parasitic infections with *Clonorchis sinensis* and *Ascaris lumbricoides*, and abnormal biliary stasis. This is a chronic disease marked by oftentimes innumerable intrahepatic pigment stones and biliary strictures, with an absence of disease within the gallbladder. Remember that key Board buzzword element—a crazy amount of stones within the biliary tree but with a normal gallbladder. Thus, the gallbladder is clearly not the origin of the stones. Instead, the stones must originate within the biliary system itself, often in the hepatic portion of the biliary system. The left hepatic system is classically affected for unclear reasons—possibly due to tighter angulations of the left ductal takeoffs compared to the right. In this case, there were innumerable stones stacked one after another up the biliary system and into the liver, as shown in Figure 76-2.

Management of acute attacks of cholangitis involves administering intravenous fluids and antibiotics, and attempts to remove as many stones as possible through ERCP. ERCP can also be used to dilate the strictures that inevitably form with recurrent attacks. Unfortunately, ERCP alone is rarely adequate, and it's often coupled with percutaneous T-tube drainage or even surgical resection of affected hepatobiliary segments. UDCA is often used, but it's probably of no real benefit for most patients because it does not effectively dissolve these calcium bilirubinate pigment stones (in contrast to its efficacy for cholesterol stones). Therapy for this complex disorder typically requires multimodal approaches including endoscopic, radiographic, and surgical therapies.

Why Might This Be Tested? Recurrent pyogenic cholangitis is a rare condition that has a nearly pathognomonic presentation.

Here's the Point!

Lots of intrahepatic and biliary pigment stones + Normal gallbladder =
Recurrent pyogenic (Oriental) cholangitis

Vignette 77: Acute Liver Failure With Super-High AST/ALT

A 59-year-old man with AIDS (CD4 count of 220) presents to the emergency room with progressive jaundice, nausea, malaise, abdominal pain, and fevers over a 1-week period. Four weeks prior to admission, he suffered a bout of severe *Pneumocystis carinii* (aka *P. jirovecii*) pneumonia, which required an inpatient hospitalization including treatment with glucocorticoids and trimethoprim-sulfamethoxazole (TMP-SMX). The patient tolerated the treatment well and eventually recovered from the illness. He was recently tested for both hepatitis B and C occult infection due to mild elevations of the AST and ALT (both 2.5 times upper limit of normal as an outpatient), with negative results. He has refused treatment with highly active antiretroviral therapy (HAART).

He now presents with 101.3°F fever in the emergency department. His exam reveals no icterus and moderate upper abdominal tenderness on palpation. The liver edge is not palpable, and there are no stigmata of chronic liver disease. There is no ascites or edema. Neurologic exam reveals hyperreflexia but no asterixis. Laboratory values include the following: WBC = 3K, hemoglobin = 12.6, platelets = 152, creatinine = 1.3, AST = 5210, ALT = 3526, ALP = 202, INR = 1.5, total bilirubin = 1.6, albumin = 3.1.

▶ **In addition to usual supportive care for acute liver injury, what other specific therapy should be considered for this patient?**

Vignette 77: Answer

You should assume this patient has acute HSV hepatitis until proven oth-erwise, and you should start acyclovir immediately due to the high mortality risk. A prompt liver biopsy (check out Figure 57-2 again) should be ordered to make the definitive diagnosis, but treatment should not be held for the results. Both HSV-1 and HSV-2 can cause run-of-the-mill hepatitis, but they can also precipitate acute liver failure. This can occur in immunocompetent people, but it should be highly considered in immunocompromised patients presenting with liver injury, such as this individual. The patient's recent exposure to steroids might have triggered this event, although it's hard to know for sure (it's generally argued that using glucocorticoids for acute pneumocystis pneumonia does not trigger opportunistic infections).

There are some clues to support HSV in this patient. First, patients with acute HSV hepatitis characteristically have very high aminotransferase levels, often in the 3000+ range, without jaundice. Second, patients with HSV hepatitis often have a relatively low white count with fever and abdominal pain—also seen in this case. Third, patients with HSV hepatitis can have coexistent HSV pneumo-nitis or encephalitis. Of course, those clues are nonspecific in and of themselves, but when coupled with the immunocompromised state and recent glucocorticoid use, you have to think of HSV.

Again, the key is to think of HSV early and start empiric acyclovir right away; don't wait to confirm HSV because it may be too late. Acute HSV hepatitis can cause acute liver failure and confers a high mortality rate. This especially holds true for pregnant women, in whom prompt treatment can often avert the need for urgent delivery if the diagnosis is made in time. Case series of HSV-induced acute liver failure consistently reveal that acyclovir is usually started too late or not at all. So the emphasis must be on early and aggressive treatment, in addition to everything else you would normally do for acute liver failure.

Why Might This Be Tested? Board examiners want to make sure you employ potentially life-saving therapies early, especially when the decision to start therapy must occur before you have a confirming diagnosis. In this case, the risk-benefit ratio of starting empiric acyclovir is overwhelmingly in favor of treatment—you just need to think about it and then take the plunge. Hesitation could spell trouble, and examiners want to know that you won't hesitate with something fundamental like this, even if the situation is uncommon.

Here's the Point!

Super-high AST/ALT without jaundice + Immunocompromised + Fever + Abdominal pain + Leukopenia = Think about acute HSV hepatitis, and start empiric acyclovir

Vignette 78: Kidney Stone and a Liver Mass

A 50-year-old man with history of nonalcoholic steatohepatitis and GERD presents with complaints of fatigue and an unintentional 20-pound weight loss over the past 3 months along with polydipsia, polyuria, and mild constipation. He mentions that he recently saw his primary care physician after he "passed a kidney stone" and had a negative evaluation for both diabetes mellitus and prostate problems. There has been no pruritus, jaundice, rigors, abdominal pain, increased abdominal girth, confusion, or memory problems. There is also no history of gastrointestinal bleeding. He reports undergoing a screening colonoscopy and upper endoscopy earlier this year that were "normal except for small veins in the esophagus." Laboratory tests reveal the following: ALT = 42, AST = 54, total bilirubin = 1.6, creatinine = 0.9, albumin = 3.4, calcium = 10.9, INR = 1.2, WBC = 3.9, hemoglobin = 12.2, platelets = 80, AFP = 108, glucose = 72, hemoglobin A_1C = 5.0%, prostate specific antigen = 1.0 ng/mL. An abdominal CT was performed, an image from which is shown in Figure 78-1. A bone scan and chest CT scan were both negative.

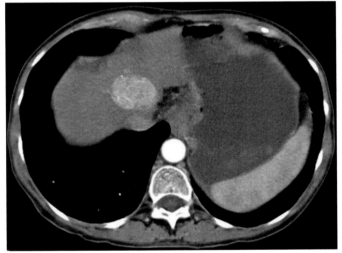

Figure 78-1. Arterial phase of triphasic abdominal CT for patient in Vignette 78. (Reprinted with permission of Barbara Kadell, MD, UCLA Medical Center.)

▶ *What is the diagnosis?*

▶ *What should you recommend?*

Vignette 78: Answer

This is hepatocellular carcinoma with a paraneoplastic syndrome due to secretion of parathyroid hormone-related protein (PTHrP) by the tumor cells. The patient has a liver mass with characteristic radiographic findings along with symptoms of hypercalcemia, including polydipsia, polyuria, constipation, and nephrolithiasis. A serum PTHrP level would be elevated if checked (normal is <1.5 pmol/L). If the patient responds to therapy for the HCC, the serum AFP, calcium, and PTHrP levels should all decrease. The lack of osteolytic lesions on bone scan essentially rules out bony metastasis as a cause of the hypercalcemia. In addition to hypercalcemia, HCC is associated with a variety of other paraneoplastic conditions related to the synthesis of active proteins. These conditions may present with symptoms and signs of erythrocytosis, hypoglycemia, diarrhea, or rashes, such as acanthosis nigricans, among other paraneoplastic phenomena.

HCC is an international public health concern; it's the fourth most common type of malignancy worldwide. In the United States, HCC is the most common primary liver cancer (metastases are the most commonly overall liver malignancy in the United States). Moreover, the incidence of HCC is expected to rise dramatically over the next 20 years due to the increase of nonalcoholic fatty liver disease and hepatitis C cirrhosis.

In patients with HCC and cirrhosis, the best outcomes with surgical resection occur with well-preserved liver function; namely, a total bilirubin level ≤1.0 and absence of advanced portal hypertension, meaning an HVPG of 10 or less. Since this patient has evidence of portal hypertension (esophageal varices on upper endoscopy along with hypersplenism) and a total bilirubin >1.0, orthotopic liver transplantation (OLT) should be considered. If the HCC characteristics fit within the Milan criteria (Table 78-1), then OLT has a 5-year survival rate of greater than 70%, which is comparable to other indications for OLT. Therefore, UNOS has adopted the Milan criteria for allocation and prioritization for OLT in HCC and assigns an initial MELD score of 22 for patients with HCC that meet the criteria. For the patient in this vignette, a MELD score of 22 would lead to a decreased waiting time on the transplant list, since his intrinsic MELD score is considerably lower (you should be able to tell this by "eyeballing" the labs, even if you have not memorized the MELD regression equation). Unfortunately, the time to OLT may

Table 78-1.
MILAN CRITERIA FOR LIVER TRANSPLANTATION
1. One lesion ≤5 cm
2. Up to 3 lesions, all ≤3 cm
3. No vascular invasion
4. No distant metastases

be prolonged (depending upon the particular region's waiting list), and patients with HCC can develop tumor progression while awaiting transplant. Therefore, if transplant is unlikely to occur within 6 months, locoregional therapy is often recommended (either radiofrequency ablation [RFA] or transarterial chemoembolization [TACE]) as a "bridge" for the patient while awaiting transplantation.

The choice of RFA versus TACE usually depends on local expertise. However, RFA is generally used for smaller lesions that do not involve the dome of the liver due to risk of tumor seeding, which is thought to be approximately 3%. TACE of feeding arteries is typically used for larger lesions as long as there is adequate hepatic reserve, since there is an increased risk for hepatic failure with TACE versus RFA; this is especially true if there is concomitant portal vein thrombosis. Remember that TACE uses the hepatic artery, and if there is a portal vein thrombosis, you essentially can cut off all significant blood supply to a large part of the liver. This may very well lead to rapid deterioration of hepatic function and death. So, you need to select the appropriate therapy on an individual basis.

Investigators have shown that if the tumor burden exceeds the Milan criteria, locoregional therapy can be used for some select tumors for "downstaging" prior to OLT. However, these patients require at least a 3-month hold to ensure that biologically favorable tumors (which have shown response to therapy) are selected for OLT.

If OLT is not possible, then locoregional therapy should be offered depending on the tumor burden and hepatic reserve. For those patients with extrahepatic metastases and/or large tumor burden who are not candidates for locoregional therapy, sorafenib (a tyrosine kinase inhibitor) can prolong survival, provided that the patient has a good performance status and adequate hepatic synthetic function. For terminal-stage patients with markedly deteriorating physical status, comfort care is recommended to avoid undue suffering.

In passing, it's worth noting other conditions, besides HCC, that are associated with an elevated AFP level. These include cholangiocarcinoma (which is also more common in patients with cirrhosis), some gastrointestinal metastatic tumors, pregnancy (yes, there it is again!), and gonadal tumors. Because elevated AFP can occur in conditions other than HCC, the diagnosis of HCC should not rely too heavily on AFP levels. Guidelines suggest diagnosing HCC on the basis of imaging and/or histology; AFP levels are now relatively de-emphasized in the diagnostic algorithm (although an AFP level of over 200 ng/mL remains highly suspicious for HCC in a patient with cirrhosis).

To diagnosis HCC without a biopsy (to avoid the risk of tumor seeding), a contrast-enhanced study is needed to show a ≥2 cm lesion with specific imaging characteristics. This can include either a triphasic CT scan or an MRI. HCC enhances more intensely than the surrounding hepatic parenchyma in the arterial phase (see Figure 78-1) and less than the surrounding liver in the venous phase, producing the "washout" appearance. If the patient in this vignette did not have a lesion on abdominal imaging, testicular ultrasound could have been performed to rule out testicular cancer as a cause of the elevated AFP.

Why might this be tested? HCC is a major health concern with a continued projected increase over the coming years. Therefore, you will encounter HCC more often and will need to know how to diagnosis and treat patients with this type of lesion, especially as therapies continue to evolve. It is also important to recognize that paraneoplastic syndromes are associated with HCC.

Clinical Threshold Alert: Patients within Milan criteria (see Table 78-1) receive an automatic MELD score of 22 independent of other MELD parameters. If OLT is unlikely for 6 months or more, then locoregional bridge therapy is warranted.

Here's the Point!

Hypercalcemia + Cirrhosis + Liver lesion + Elevated AFP =
Hepatocellular carcinoma with elevated PTHrP

Vignettes 79 to 86: Liver Histology Throw-Down

You are probably not a pathologist. But for purposes of the Board exam, you will need know a slew of pathology buzzwords to navigate through many of the questions. This collection of mini-vignettes provides a set of classic pathology buzzwords with minimal surrounding information. Most of these diagnoses are featured elsewhere in this book along with characteristic micrographs. However, the buzzwords alone may be enough for you to determine the diagnosis. Read each vignette, and then make the diagnosis. By the way, we thought the "owl's eye" intranuclear inclusion finding was too much of a gimme. You remember that one, right? If not, better go back to Figure 57-1.

79. An obese patient undergoes liver biopsy for persistently elevated aminotransferase levels. The AST:ALT ratio has always been less than 1.0. Liver biopsy reveals steatosis with lobular infiltration and ballooning hepatocytes.

80. A patient with cholestasis has a liver biopsy revealing a "florid duct lesion" marked by bile duct destruction, "ductopenia," and granulomas.

81. A patient with cholestasis has a liver biopsy revealing periductal "onion-skinning fibrosis."

82. A patient with elevated transaminases and an elevated gamma globulin has interface hepatitis with a plasma cell infiltrate and lobular inflammation on liver biopsy.

83. Nutmeg liver (yep, that's all you get).

84. A patient with elevated transaminases has PAS-positive diastase-resistant globules in hepatocytes on liver biopsy.

85. A patient with long-standing elevations in AST and ALT has "ground-glass hepatocytes" on liver biopsy.

86. A former intravenous drug user is referred to you for persistently elevated liver enzymes (AST = 89, ALT = 110) and transferrin saturation (85%). Recent liver biopsy revealed the presence of hemosiderin in Kupffer cells but not in hepatocytes.

Vignettes 79 to 86: Answers

79. This is NASH. Clinical clues include obesity and the AST:ALT ratio below 1.0 (whereas alcoholic liver disease typically has a ratio above 2.0). See Vignette 37 for more information on NASH and NAFLD. Board buzzwords for NASH include lobular inflammation, ballooning hepatocytes, and portal inflammation. Other features include Mallory bodies, fibrosis, and ultimately cirrhosis (Figure 79-1).

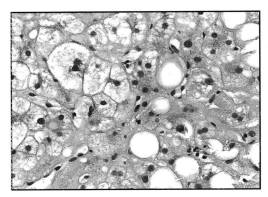

Figure 79-1. Nonalcoholic steatohepatitis with ballooning hepatocytes. (Reprinted with permission of Alton B. Farris, MD, Emory University.)

Here's the Point!

NASH Histopathology Board Buzzwords:
- **Lobular inflammation**
- **Ballooning hepatocytes**
- **Portal inflammation**
- **Mallory bodies**

80. This is primary biliary cirrhosis. PBC is a progressive, destructive disease that decimates the bile ducts over time. Early on, it produces a so-called florid duct lesion marked by bile duct destruction, a severe lymphoplasmacytic infiltrate in the portal tracts, and granulomas. Refer to Vignette 35 and Figure 35-1 for more information about PBC, and to Vignette 56 for information on the PBC overlap syndrome with autoimmune hepatitis.

Here's the Point!

High ALP + Florid duct lesion + Granulomas = PBC

81. This is primary sclerosing cholangitis. PSC can sometimes produce a similar appearance to PBC, but it's not associated with granulomas. Instead, the classic feature of PSC is a fibrous obliterative cholangitis that looks like "onion skinning" around the bile ducts, as shown in Figure 81-1 (although any condition with chronic duct obstruction can cause onion-skinning fibrosis). Both PBC and PSC can lead to "ductopenia" or to a lack of bile ducts altogether in the burnt-out stage.

Figure 81-1. Primary sclerosing cholangitis with "onion-skinning" obliterative fibrosis on trichrome staining. (Reprinted with permission of Charles Lassman, MD, UCLA Medical Center.)

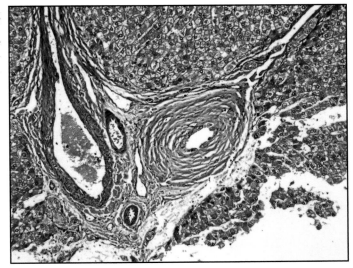

Here's the Point!

High ALP + Onion skinning = Think PSC

82. This is autoimmune hepatitis. AIH is classically associated with elevated transaminases in association with elevated gamma globulin levels. Characteristic histologic changes include interface hepatitis with a plasma cell infiltrate (Figure 82-1). In particular, the limiting plate of the portal tract is invaded by the infiltrating plasma cells, which, in turn, extend into the lobule.

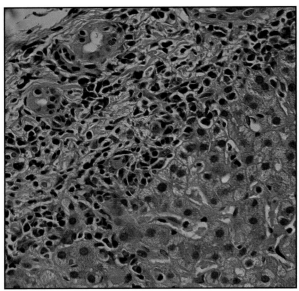

Figure 82-1. Autoimmune hepatitis with plasma cell infiltrate and interface hepatitis. (Reprinted with permission of Charles Lassman, MD, UCLA Medical Center.)

Here's the Point!

Interface hepatitis + Plasma cell infiltrate = Autoimmune hepatitis

83. This is congestive hepatopathy. The term *nutmeg liver* is a fanciful one, sort of like many terms cooked up by pathologists who spend too much time looking through microscopes in a sub-sub basement. "Nutmeg" refers to the speckled appearance of the liver from passive congestion; evidently this looks something like a grated nutmeg kernel on gross examination. Microscopically, there are dark areas from dilated hepatic venules that are full of blood, and light areas that are unaffected surrounding parenchyma (Figure 83-1). Nutmeg liver most commonly results from right-sided heart failure or Budd-Chiari syndrome.

Figure 83-1. Congestive hepatopathy. (Reprinted with permission of Charles Lassman, MD, UCLA Medical Center.)

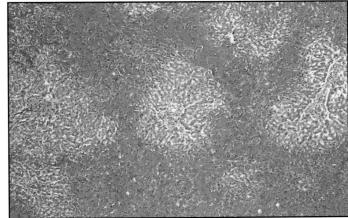

Here's the Point!

Nutmeg liver = Congestive hepatopathy from right-heart failure or Budd-Chiari syndrome

84. This is alpha-1 antitrypsin (A1AT) deficiency. A1AT deficiency is an autosomal codominant disorder that leads to a range of problems, including liver disease, pulmonary emphysema, panniculitis, and arterial aneurysms. The liver manifestations of A1AT deficiency arise from a defect in protein secretion from the endoplasmic reticulum. The A1AT proteins get "stuck" and accumulate in the hepatocyte endoplasmic reticulum, and are classically detected as PAS-positive "globules" that are "diastase resistant" (Figure 84.1).

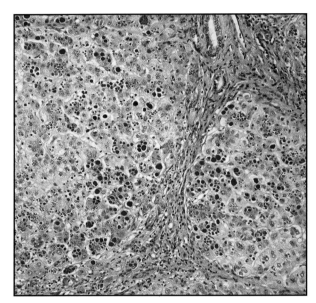

Figure 84-1. A1AT deficiency with PAS stain demonstrating "diastase-resistant" intrahepatic globules. (Reprinted with permission of Charles Lassman, MD, UCLA Medical Center.)

Here's the Point!

**PAS-positive diastase-resistant gobules in Hepatocytes =
Alpha-1 antitrypsin (A1AT) deficiency**

85. This is chronic infection with hepatitis B virus. Ground-glass hepatocytes are a hallmark of HBV infection. *Ground glass* is another fanciful term from a weary pathologist that describes the hazy and dull appearance of hepatocyte cytoplasm in chronic HBV infection (Figure 85-1). The ground glass is composed of surface antigens (sAg) from the HBV; the surface antigens collect in the endoplasmic reticulum of the hepatocytes to create this visual effect on microscopy. The ground-glass appearance does not occur in acute HBV—only chronic HBV. Ground-glass hepatocytes also have been described in some other conditions (eg, drug induced, Lafora disease, fibrinogen storage disease, type IV glycogenosis), but HBV is by far the most common cause.

Figure 85-1. Hepatitis B virus with ground-glass hepatocytes. (Reprinted with permission of Charles Lassman, MD, UCLA Medical Center.)

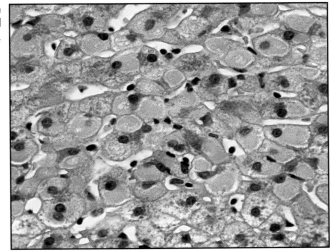

Here's the Point!

Ground-glass hepatocytes = Chronic infection with hepatitis B virus

86. This is hemosiderosis, probably from underlying chronic viral hepatitis. The key here is to distinguish hemochromatosis from hemosiderosis. The former leads to iron deposition in the hepatocytes, and the latter leads to iron deposition in the Kupffer cells, which are the macrophages of the liver. Both can be associated with an elevated transferrin saturation. Hemochromatosis may lead to transaminase elevations, but hemosiderosis, in and of itself, is less likely to cause transaminases to rise to 3 times the upper limit of normal, as occurred here. So we need to posit an underlying condition that can lead to both hemosiderosis and transaminemia. There are 3 common liver conditions that fit the bill: chronic viral hepatitis, nonalcoholic fatty liver disease, and alcoholic liver disease. This former intravenous drug user is at risk for viral hepatitis, in particular, so that should be high on the differential diagnosis. Hemolytic anemia is the most common *non*-liver cause of secondary iron overload. Whereas phlebotomy is the standard management of hemochromatosis, it has no role in the management of hemosiderosis. Iron chelation therapy is often used in patients with hemosiderosis due to hemolytic anemia, but this is not typically a decision overseen by a hepatologist or gastroenterologist.

Here's the Point!

Iron in hepatocytes = Hemochromatosis
Iron in Kupffer cells = Hemosiderosis

Vignette 87: Genetic Variations in Hepatitis C Treatment Response

Chronic infection with HCV is currently treated with combination therapy using pegylated interferon-alpha (peg-IFN-alfa) and ribavirin (RBV). Treatment responses are especially low in genotype 1 HCV (around 45%) as compared to genotypes 2 and 3 HCV. Moreover, the genotype 1 SVR is usually lower in patients of African ancestry compared to the SVR in those of European or Asian ancestry. A recent biological discovery has revealed a major genetic reason why responses to IFN and RBV vary so much by ethnicity.

▶ *What is the reason?*

Vignette 87: Answer

Ethnic variations in treatment response are partly determined by genetic polymorphisms near the interleukin-28B (IL-28B) gene, which encodes interferon-lambda-3 (IFN-λ-3). You may think this is too arcane to show up on a Board exam, but it's not. This topic is prime time, and there is no time like the present to understand this fascinating biological story with immediate clinical implications.

So what's the deal here? It is known that Caucasians and Asians tend to have better treatment response rates for HCV than Latinos or people of African descent, and there is now a commercially available test that can predict nearly half the variation in HCV treatment response rates between these patients of different ancestry. This test is based on the results of several genome-wide association studies that have found a single nucleotide polymorphism (SNP) just upstream from the IL-28B gene on chromosome 19 that significantly affects response rates to peg-INF-alfa and RBV. As noted, the IL-28B gene normally codes for IFN-λ-3 (the "lambda form" of interferon), which has its own antiviral activity. So if this intrinsic interferon is not produced as a consequence of a genetic polymorphism of the gene, then the treatment effect of peg-IFN-alfa and RBV will be undermined. The polymorphism consists of CC, CT, and TT genotypes of IL-28B. The CC genotype leads to higher levels of IFN-λ-3 production. In contrast, the CT and TT genotypes lead to lower levels of IFN-λ-3 production. Those patients with the CC genotype have a 2-fold higher response rate to peg-IFN-alfa and RBV than those with the CT and TT genotypes. And the CC genotype is much more common in patients of Asian and European ancestry, whereas it's less prevalent in patients of African and Latino ancestry.

This is pretty fascinating, but it's also clinically relevant. It has been shown that the presence of the CC IL-28B genotype predicts >2-fold rate of RVR, complete EVR, and SVR compared to the presence of the CT and TT IL-28 genotypes (recall the details on the basic viral kinetics of HCV from Vignette 64). Furthermore, in those patients who did not achieve an RVR, the CC genotype also had a >2-fold increase in achieving an SVR compared with the CT and TT genotypes. Because treatment for genotype 1 HCV is extremely expensive, onerous, and rife with adverse events, knowing a patient's IL-28B genotype might help to make or break the decision to treat. As mentioned earlier, if a patient has the favorable CC genotype, then treatment is much more likely to work. If the patient does not have this genotype, the likelihood of achieving an SVR is considerably lower, especially if there are other factors undermining success (discussed more later in this vignette). In fact, the IL-28B polymorphism is the most potent pretreatment predictor of SVR in genotype 1 patients. Of course, achieving an RVR is the strongest overall predictor for attaining an SVR.

Recently, the fight against HCV got a lot more interesting with the arrival of direct acting anti-viral agents (DAAs) previously called specifically targeted anti-viral therapy for HCV (STAT-C). Two linear protease inhibitors (PIs) directed against the NS3/4a protease (telaprevir and boceprevir) are approved for use in a combination "triple therapy" regimen (peg-IFN-alpha + RBV + PI) for genotype 1 HCV. This triple therapy regimen has improved SVR rates and can shorten the treatment period. However, there are increased drug interactions and side effects, including rash and anemia, in particular. Furthermore, the development of resistance can blow it for an entire class of DAAs. For this reason, the same class of PIs should not be used together or as monotherapy and vigilance is required to monitor for lack of response or virological breakthrough. Data is accumulating in regards to the IL-28 genotype and DAA triple therapy to help prognosticate SVR rates further. Get ready for even more DAAs, since polymerase inhibitors and cyclophilin inhibitors will be joining the armamentarium in the years to come!

While we are on the topic of predicting treatment response in HCV, it's worth listing other clinical factors known to adversely impact the efficacy of INF and RBV. These include higher baseline viral load, higher age, male sex, higher body mass index, presence of insulin resistance, hepatic steatosis, and hepatic fibrosis. We know genotypes 2 and 3 have much higher rates of response than genotype 1 HCV. In addition, genotype 2 tends to have a higher treatment response than genotype 3. Furthermore, genotype 3 is associated with steatosis, which tends to improve with treatment.

Why Might This Be Tested? This story is so biologically interesting, and the IL-28B genotype is such a strong predictor of SVR, that it's hard to imagine this won't show up on an exam soon. The availability of a commercially available test makes this a clinically relevant discovery. And this polymorphism explains much of the variance in response between patients of different ancestry. You probably will not need to know too much about this polymorphism, other than it exists and what it's called.

Here's the Point!

Genetic polymorphisms in IL-28B significantly predict treatment success from peg-INF-alfa and RBV in chronic HCV. This polymorphism also explains over half the variation in treatment differences between patients of different ancestry.

Vignette 88: More Swelling

A 59-year-old man with HCV cirrhosis complains of increased fatigue and dyspnea with minimal exertion over the past several months. He has been compliant with sodium restriction and increasing diuretic therapy but has had "more swelling" in his abdomen and legs. There is no history of smoking. Physical examination is notable for muscle wasting, marked ascites, and pedal edema. His lungs are clear to auscultation, and he is noted to have a loud P2 heart sound with jugular venous distention and a high-pitched holosystolic murmur at the lower left sternal border accentuated with inspiration. There is no cyanosis.

▶ **What is the diagnosis? (That's right, you don't need any labs or imaging.)**

Vignette 88: Answer

This is portopulmonary hypertension (PPHTN). The history and physical examination should clue you in to the diagnosis before you even look at labs or imaging. In addition to the accentuation of the tricuspid regurgitant murmur, physical exam may also reveal an increased right ventricular heave with inspiration. An echocardiogram may show right ventricular hypertrophy with elevated pulmonary artery pressures. However, the gold standard for diagnosis is to perform a right heart catheterization with hemodynamic measurements. Of course, further imaging, laboratory testing, and cardiopulmonary tests would be helpful to rule out other etiologies for this patient's clinical deterioration.

Cirrhosis, by itself, causes a hyperdynamic circulation and a volume overloaded state, which can cause a minimal increase in pulmonary artery pressures. However, when there is increased pulmonary vascular resistance due to PPHTN, this will lead to marked increases in pulmonary artery pressures. To confirm the diagnosis, a right heart catheterization would need to show a resting mean pulmonary artery pressure (MPAP) >25 mm Hg and an increased pulmonary vascular resistance (PVR) >240 dynes/s/cm^{-5} with a pulmonary capillary wedge pressure (PCWP) <15 mm Hg.

PPHTN has a poor prognosis with median survival of approximately 15 months. Several treatments have been used in PPHTN including prostacyclin, phosphodiesterase inhibitors, endothelin receptor antagonists, oxygen, and anticoagulation. However, liver transplantation provides the best option in select patients with mild PPHTN whose MPAP can fall below 35 mm Hg with medical therapy, provided that right heart function is also deemed acceptable. Although PPHTN occurs in up to 15% of patients undergoing evaluation for liver transplantation, the severity of PPHTN does not correlate well with the MELD score. Therefore, exception MELD scores often can be given to these patients if they are approved for transplant. Liver transplantation is not generally offered to patients with MPAP >35 mm Hg due to the high perioperative risk.

Why Might This Be Tested? The history and physical examination alone (as provided in this vignette) are critical to decide which further tests to order to ascertain this diagnosis. Board examiners love to throw in cardiac physical examination findings; PPHTN represents a perfect clinical scenario to test your knowledge.

Clinical Threshold Alert:
1. 25 mm Hg is the minimum MPAP for diagnosis.
2. 35 mm Hg is the maximum MPAP for liver transplant consideration.

Here's the Point!

Cirrhosis + Loud P2 + Tricuspid regurgitation + Increased edema →
Think PPHTN

Vignettes 89 to 92: More Pregnancy Woes

The following mini-vignettes describe liver diseases that are unique to pregnancy. See if you can determine the diagnosis for each one using the minimal information provided.

89. A 21-year-old nulliparous woman presents with severe nausea, vomiting, and fatigue at 8 weeks' gestation. She has had no fever, diarrhea, or ill contacts. Labs include the following: ALT = 340, AST = 290, total bilirubin = 1.9, WBC = 6.5, hemoglobin = 14.8, platelets = 271, glucose = 78, INR = 1.0, and creatinine = 1.3.

90. A 36-year-old nulliparous woman, who is expecting twins via in vitro fertilization, presents with pruritus leading to insomnia at 28 weeks' gestation. The pruritus started on her palms and soles, and now she describes having to "scratch myself to death." Labs include the following: ALT = 56, AST = 51, total bilirubin = 1.4, WBC = 6.1, hemoglobin = 12.8, platelets = 204, glucose = 90, INR = 1.7, and creatinine = 0.8.

91. A 28-year-old nulliparous woman at 36 weeks' gestation presents with malaise, nausea, vomiting, epigastric pain, and jaundice but no fever. Her husband mentions that she has been sleeping most of the day. Labs include the following: ALT = 298, ALT = 268, total bilirubin = 4.9, WBC = 14.8, hemoglobin = 10.9, platelets = 140, glucose = 59, INR = 2.1, and creatinine = 1.7.

92. A 29-year-old multiparous woman at 31 weeks' gestation presents with worsening fatigue, edema, headache, nausea, and vomiting without fever. However, she now has severe, unrelenting abdominal pain and feels lightheaded. There is no melena, hematochezia, hematemesis, or vaginal bleeding. Labs include the following: ALT = 166, AST = 190, total bilirubin = 3.8, WBC = 8.2, hemoglobin = 6.7, platelets = 63, glucose = 80, INR = 1.3, and creatinine = 1.6.

Vignettes 89 to 92: Answers

89. This is hyperemesis gravidarum (HG). HG occurs early in pregnancy, usually at 4 to 10 weeks' gestation (first trimester), and almost always resolves by week 20. The exact etiology of HG remains unknown, but several factors have been studied. A classic fact is that liver biopsy reveals little or no pathology. Inpatient supportive care with antiemetics, intravenous fluids, vitamin replacement, and bowel rest is recommended. This clinical picture closely resembles acute viral hepatitis, which needs to be excluded. Urinalysis and right upper quadrant ultrasound are also important to exclude pyelonephritis and gallstone-related disease, respectively. The maternal and fetal prognosis for HG is excellent.

90. This is intrahepatic cholestasis of pregnancy (ICP), which is the second leading cause of jaundice in pregnancy (you know the first, right?). The diagnostic test of choice is serum bile acids, which can be elevated up to 100-fold and clinches the diagnosis. Higher bile acid levels (especially more than 40 µmol/L) in ICP carry an increased risk of complications. ICP usually occurs in the third trimester but may sometimes present at the end of the second trimester. Risk factors for the development of ICP include having multiple pregnancies, multiple gestations, and being of advanced age. Furthermore, there is a genetic predisposition for developing ICP, and it's more common in certain populations, including persons of Chilean descent. Physical examination may reveal diffuse excoriations. Although the maternal outcome is good, this is not a benign condition for the fetus. There is a significant fetal risk for premature delivery, fetal distress, meconium ileus, and stillbirth, with up to a 4% mortality. Furthermore, there tends to be subclinical steatorrhea associated with the cholestasis, which can lead to vitamin K deficiency (causing the elevated INR) in the mother and fetus. Vitamin K replacement can reduce the risk of postpartum hemorrhage, which can be quite severe. Patients with ICP may also develop cholelithiasis. Treatment with ursodeoxycholic acid (13 to 15 mg/kg/day) is helpful to minimize the symptoms, and prompt delivery is recommended if there is any sign of fetal distress. ICP tends to recur in more than half of future pregnancies, so patients need to be informed of this risk before getting pregnant again. Oh, and what is the most common cause of jaundice in pregnancy? Right, viral hepatitis.

91. This is acute fatty liver of pregnancy (AFLP), which means trouble! AFLP is quite rare to encounter in real life, occurring in 1 in 10,000 deliveries, but is much more common on Board exams! The etiology stems from impairments of intramitochondrial fatty acid oxidation, sometimes involving a mutation causing long-chain 3-hydroxyacyl-coenzyme A dehydrogenase (LCHAD) deficiency. In fact, approximately 20% of newborns of women with AFLP will have homozygous LCHAD deficiency. The inability of the fetus to oxidize long-chain fatty acids causes these acids to accumulate in the maternal circulation via placental transfer. The heterozygous mother, in turn, has a reduced capacity to oxidize these long-chain fatty acids, which leads to the microvesicular steatosis, encephalopathy, and liver failure in the mother during the third trimester. If the diagnosis is unclear, urgent liver biopsy is needed on fresh specimen using oil red O staining to examine for microvesicular steatosis (Figure 91-1). Both maternal mortality and fetal mortality are up to 20%. Thus, prompt diagnosis and delivery are mandated. Furthermore, vigilant intensive care monitoring is necessary for the mother after delivery. If recovery is not swift, the patient should be urgently referred to a liver transplant center for transplant evaluation. To compound matters, the newborn with LCHAD deficiency is at risk for potentially fatal, fasting nonketotic hypoglycemia over the next several months. Therefore, it's mandatory to check the newborn for LCHAD deficiency. The risk of recurrence is low with future pregnancies, but most women choose not to get pregnant again after AFLP (which is not terribly shocking after going through the ordeal).

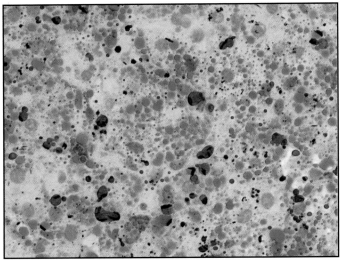

Figure 91-1. Acute fatty liver of pregnancy with oil red O stain showing the microvesicular fatty infiltration in the hepatocytes. (Reprinted with permission of Charles Lassman, MD, UCLA Medical Center.)

92. This is HELLP (Hemolysis, Elevated LFTs, and Low Platelets) syndrome complicated by hepatic rupture, which is another obstetric emergency! HELLP occurs within the setting of pre-eclampsia in some cases (a great deal more often than AFLP does). Thus, hypertension, proteinuria, and edema (the classic triad of preeclampsia signs) are often present in HELLP. Of note, preeclampsia on its own merit can also cause liver necrosis in severe cases. However, with HELLP syndrome there is thrombocytopenia, an elevated LDH level, indirect hyperbilirubinemia, and low haptoglobin from the microangiopathic hemolytic anemia associated with the condition. Histologically, there is periportal hemorrhage, fibrin deposition in the sinusoids, and focal ischemic necrosis consistent with the vascular changes that occur with the condition. If there is sudden and severe abdominal pain with acutely worsened anemia, look for hepatic rupture or subcapsular hematoma, which carries a mortality rate for the mother and fetus of up to 60%. Treatment consists of prompt delivery with angiographic embolization and/or surgery to stop the bleeding. Because this disaster can also occur after delivery, intensive care monitoring of the mother is required until recovery. Preeclampsia or HELLP tends to recur in up to one third of future pregnancies.

Why Might This Be Tested? The liver disorders that are unique to pregnancy can cause significant morbidity and mortality to the mother and fetus. Therefore, it's important to diagnose these conditions accurately and efficiently. In addition, it's important to exclude other disorders that can mimic some these conditions, such as acute viral hepatitis or biliary disease, since the treatment can be quite different. These are challenges for which your obstetrics colleagues will look to you for guidance.

Clinical Threshold Alert: 13 to 15 mg/kg/day is the target range for therapeutic dosing of ursodeoxycholic acid for the treatment of ICP and PBC.

Here's the Point!

LIVER DISEASES UNIQUE TO PREGNANCY				
Condition	Trimester	Key Labs	Pathology	Approximate Incidence
Hyperemesis gravidarum	1st	None are specific	Little to none on biopsy	1 in 200
Intrahepatic cholestasis of pregnancy	2nd/ 3rd	Elevated bile acids (above 10 μmol/L)	Bland cholestasis	1 in 1000
Acute fatty liver of pregnancy	3rd or postpartum	High INR; Low glucose	Microvesicular steatosis	1 in 10,000
HELLP	3rd or postpartum	Low platelets High LDH High indirect bilirubin	Periportal hemorrhage with focal ischemic necrosis	1 in 200

Here's the Point!

ICP $\longrightarrow$ **High recurrence rate and is not a benign condition for the fetus**

Here's the Point!

ICP ⟶ Increased cholelithiasis

Here's the Point!

AFLP ⟶ Microvesicular steatosis, and can progress after delivery

Here's the Point!

AFLP ⟶ Check for LCHAD deficiency in newborn to avoid fatal hypoglycemia

Here's the Point!

With HELLP, hepatic rupture or intraperitoneal bleeding can also occur after delivery.

Vignette 93: PSC in UC

A 51-year-old woman with chronic, progressive ulcerative colitis undergoes total colectomy after lack of response to medical therapy. There is no history of PSC, and her ALP and GGT levels have been normal. She had read about PSC and now wants to know if the colectomy will protect her from developing PSC in the future.

▶ *Has the colectomy removed her risk of developing PSC?*

Vignette 93: Answer

No. Unfortunately, colectomy does not remove the risk of developing PSC in patients with UC. It is important to recognize, however, that the overall risk of developing PSC in UC is low, regardless of colectomy. Case series reveal that up to 7.5% of UC patients develop PSC. The converse is not true. That is, patients with PSC are at much higher risk of developing UC; up to 80% of PSC patients are ultimately diagnosed with UC. Moreover, liver transplant does not remove the risk of developing UC. For this reason patients with PSC should undergo routine surveillance colonoscopy as if they are in a high-risk group for colorectal cancer, even if they have had a liver transplant; they may already harbor underlying colonic dysplasia even if a formal diagnosis of UC has not been established. But patients with UC need not undergo routine MRCP or ERCP to screen for PSC unless there is some clinical indication of PSC, such as an elevated ALP, GGT, or bilirubin level.

The relationship between UC and PSC is pretty complicated. For example, UC patients with PSC have a higher risk of colorectal cancer than UC patients without PSC. In fact, PSC is an independent risk factor for colorectal cancer, although the reason is unclear. The risk of colorectal cancer is especially high in patients who have had UC for at least 10 years and who also have PSC. Another curious fact is that compared to UC patients without PSC, those with PSC have a higher incidence of pouchitis following total colectomy with ileal pouch–anal anastomosis. And the pouchitis will persist even if they undergo liver transplant for the PSC.

Why Might This Be Tested? Board examiners have a number of content "check boxes" they need to check off when putting an exam together. This topic is convenient because it covers several areas, including hepatobiliary disorders, luminal pathology, and even liver transplant. With one question they could potentially test across several content areas.

Here's the Point!

> **Colectomy does not protect against developing PSC in UC.**
> **Liver transplant does not protect against developing UC in PSC.**

Vignette 94: Stones

A 40-year-old obese woman at 18 weeks' gestation presents with intermittent bouts of postprandial epigastric abdominal pain, nausea, and vomiting for the past few weeks. Her latest episode was quite severe prompting her to come in to the emergency department. She is admitted to the hospital with the following labs: creatinine = 1.0, total bilirubin = 1.3, AST = 76, ALT = 38, ALP = 130, lipase = 1658, WBC = 11.8, and hemoglobin = 14.2. An abdominal ultrasound shows multiple gallstones in the gallbladder without thickening or pericholecystic fluid noted. The common bile duct is reported as normal and 4 mm in diameter; pancreatic views are obscured by bowel artifact. She receives intravenous fluids and analgesia by the obstetrics service. You are consulted the next day and note that her pain and nausea have resolved completely. The patient wants to know when she can eat, since she has been placed on *nil per os* status. She feels well now and wants to go home. She states that she will follow up with you as an outpatient if she has abdominal pain again. Her obstetrician told her that discharge home today would be fine if it were approved by the GI service. Her laboratory tests today include the following: creatinine = 0.7, total bilirubin = 1.0, AST = 32, ALT = 28, ALP = 128, lipase = 430, WBC = 8.4, hemoglobin = 13.1, platelets = 210.

▶ *Should you agree with the patient's plan?*

Vignette 94: Answer

No to this one, too. This patient has recovered from gallstone pancreatitis and should now have a surgical consult for laparoscopic cholecystectomy. She requires timely surgical treatment; delay in treatment carries significant morbidity to the fetus and mother if there is a recurrent episode. Therefore, it would *not* be appropriate to follow her expectantly. You should advise against her plan and should recommend that she not be discharged home without a cholecystectomy. It was previously thought that cholecystectomy should be performed only in the second trimester due to concerns of fetal demise in the first trimester and induction of premature labor in the third trimester. However, immediate cholecystectomy should be considered whenever there is severe acute cholecystitis not responding to conservative management, intractable biliary colic, or gallstone pancreatitis. In these scenarios, there would be too much risk for both the fetus and mother with delay. Board examinations tend to avoid questions regarding areas of controversy, which is why this question described a patient in her second trimester of pregnancy. Nonetheless, *any* pregnant patient with uncomplicated symptomatic biliary colic should have a cholecystectomy, ideally in the second trimester if possible. Of note, the laparoscopic approach involves less uterine irritation and less postoperative analgesia and is favored over the open approach.

ERCP with sphincterotomy can be performed if there is choledocholithiasis. Of course, care should be taken to minimize the fluoroscopy time, and the fetus must be covered with a protective shield. In addition to the total amount of radiation exposure, the timing of radiation is of utmost importance. The first week of gestation is the most risky time to get irradiated (however, most women don't even know they are pregnant during this time).

Cholelithiasis is prevalent in pregnant women (about 10%) due to estrogen increasing cholesterol synthesis and increased gallbladder volumes. This promotes biliary lithogenicity; however, less than 1% have symptomatic cholelithiasis. Gallstones need to be considered in the workup of abdominal pain in the pregnant patient. By the way, this patient fits the (not politically correct) 4 F's of gallstones that we all learned in medical school: Female, Fertile, Forty, and Fat.

Why Might This Be Tested? Gallstones are common in pregnancy, and symptomatic disease will often prompt a consult to a gastroenterologist for management (before the surgery consult). Everybody will be looking to you to provide answers. So you need to recommend wisely.

Here's the Point!

Cholecystectomy for complicated biliary colic during pregnancy should not be delayed.

Here's the Point!

Uncomplicated biliary colic should prompt laparoscopic cholecystectomy (preferably in the second trimester).

Vignette 95: Cough and an Elevated ALP

A 68-year-old Mexican-American presents to his primary care provider for management of a chronic cough. During the course of his workup, laboratories reveal abnormal liver tests including ALP = 234, AST = 99, ALT = 67, and total bilirubin = 1.4. He is referred to you for further evaluation. On questioning, you learn that he lived on a farm growing up where he prepared wool from sheep. He immigrated to the United States when he was 35. He does not drink alcohol. He does not have a history of liver disease. Although he has had a chronic cough for several months, he does not smoke. He is febrile on examination. His liver is enlarged, spanning 15 cm, and is not tender. There are no other stigmata of chronic liver disease. The rest of his examination is unremarkable. Testing for amebiasis is negative.

▸ **What is the most likely diagnosis?**

▸ **What is the best way to confirm this diagnosis?**

Vignette 95: Answer

This is most likely an echinococcal (aka "hydatid") cyst of the liver. Echinococcal liver cysts occur from chronic infection with the *Echinococcus granulosus* tapeworm. This tapeworm is especially prevalent in South and Central America, the Middle East, China, and Sub-Saharan Africa. The life cycle is complex and involves sheep and dogs, so the classic Board buzzword here is "sheepherder." When you hear about a sheepherder, think about echinococcosis and fascioliasis (see Vignette 44). This patient was not a sheepherder, but he certainly hung around sheep. In any event, humans are an accidental host in the echinococcal life cycle. Echinococcosis can exist in humans for years without causing symptoms, only to show up years later in the form of pulmonary disease or liver cysts, among many other manifestations. So the other clue in a Board question is hearing about a cough along with some liver trouble. Cough plus liver trouble can be many things (eg, sarcoidosis, alpha-1 antitrypsin deficiency, coccidioidomycosis), but cough with a high ALP in someone from Central America should also make you think about an echinococcal cyst, in particular. Any space-filling lesion of the liver can cause the ALP to be elevated out of proportion to the other liver tests; echinococcal cysts are no exception.

When *E. granulosus* infects the liver, it tends to most commonly affect the right lobe. This distribution is common among liver infections, since the right lobe is larger and receives more of the mesenteric vessel drainage than other parts of the liver. So keep this clue in mind when reading Board vignettes about liver lesions. The echinococcal liver cysts are often totally asymptomatic and only detected through biochemical abnormalities, as seen here. However, once the cysts grow large, they can cause trouble; this typically occurs when the cysts expand to more than 10 cm in diameter. Once the cyst becomes large, it leads to hepatomegaly (as seen here) and may cause abdominal pain or discomfort from stretching of the liver capsule. In severe cases, the cyst can rupture into the biliary system and trigger a number of problems including biliary obstruction, cholangitis, or even pancreatitis. The cyst can also compress local vessels including the portal vein, hepatic vein, and inferior vena cava. When this occurs the patient can present with portal hypertension, Budd-Chiari syndrome, or venous obstruction with lower extremity edema.

The next step in this case is to confirm the diagnosis. Diagnosing echinococcal cysts may include both imaging and serologic studies (echinococcal antibodies), although the imaging is usually done first. Ultrasound is highly sensitive for detecting these cysts and is often employed as the first diagnostic study. The ultrasonographic appearance is classically a smooth, round cyst with "daughter cysts" and internal septations. These cysts can be calcified and have an "eggshell" appearance due to the calcified wall—another classic Board buzzword. These cysts may also contain so-called hydatid sand, which consists of various parts of the tapeworms themselves (literally, the hooks and scolices of the tapeworm form a granulated, sand-like substance within the cyst). Detailed sonographic characteristics can be used to classify these cysts as active, transitional, or inactive, and the classification has treatment implications, as will be described shortly. CT scanning can reveal the same basic information but with even better accuracy (Figure 95-1), and is often used for monitoring cyst size over time.

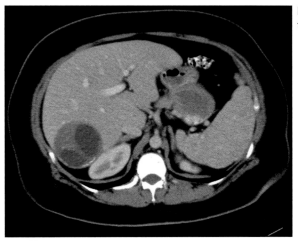

Figure 95-1. Typical echinoccocal liver cyst in the right lobe of the liver.

Sometimes it's hard to confirm the diagnosis because the imaging is ambiguous, the serology is negative, or both. In such cases percutaneous cyst aspiration can be used to obtain fluid to evaluate for the worms themselves. This is where distinguishing active from inactive cysts is helpful; active cysts are under high pressure, whereas inactive cysts are not. The most worrisome consequence of aspiration is triggering an anaphylactic reaction to the spilled cyst contents. This is rare but can be devastating.

As a random aside, an earlier vignette involved cysts that fill up with so-called anchovy paste (another Board buzzword). Are these the same type of cysts? The answer is no; anchovy paste is described in abscesses from *Entamoeba histolytica* (see Vignette 38). This patient also tested negative for amebiasis. Table 44-1 contains Board buzzword associations regarding liver parasites. That table contains a gold mine of information for the Board exam.

Treatment of echinococcal cysts depends upon several factors and may include a combination of albendazole, repeated percutaneous aspirations, and surgery. Surgery is employed when the cysts are really large (ie, ≥10 cm), complex, or near the capsule and at risk of rupture regardless of size. Smaller or less complicated cysts are typically treated with either albendazole or percutaneous aspirations. The details beyond this get fairly complicated and are not reviewed in depth here.

Why Might This Be Tested? This diagnosis is chock-full of Board buzzwords, so it's a perfect setup for a test question.

Clinical Threshold Alert: Echinococcal liver cyst exceeding 10 cm typically requires surgery.

Here's the Point!

Sheepherder + Central or South America + Cough + Liver cyst with septations, eggshell calcifications, and hydatid sand = Echinococcosis

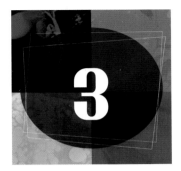

60 HEPATOLOGY BOARD REVIEW "CLINICAL THRESHOLD VALUES"

Many exam questions require that test-takers have memorized some numerical threshold value, like: *"If an echinococcal cyst exceeds XX cm, then the risk of rupture is clinically significant and surgery is warranted."* Or: *"If the ALT:LDH ratio exceeds Y:Y in the setting of severe transaminemia, then acute viral hepatitis is the most likely diagnosis."* These values have been highlighted throughout this book. What follows is a "one-stop shop" for all these numerical facts. These are presented by increasing numerical order—not by a rational taxonomy. So the resulting list will seem like a pretty random hodgepodge, which is the point. Exam questions are random too, so just go with the flow.

1.0 = If the ratio of urine sodium to potassium in a spot urine sample is greater than this value in cirrhosis (ie, more urinary Na than K), then the patient has a sufficient response to diuretic therapy and is likely to have >78 mEq Na per day during a full 24-hour urine collection.

1.1 = If the serum–ascites albumin gradient (SAAG) equals or exceeds this value, then portal hypertensive ascites is 97% likely.

1.5 = If the ALT:LDH ratio exceeds this value in the setting of severe transaminemia (eg, ALT and AST in the 1000+ range), then acute viral hepatitis is likely. If the ratio is lower than this value, consider drug-induced, toxin-induced, or hypoxemic-induced liver injury.

2 = If the AST:ALT ratio exceeds this value in the setting of biochemical hepatitis, and assuming the ALT is below 500 U/L, then alcoholic liver injury is likely. Of note, cirrhosis due to any cause can also have this ratio, but typically with lower transaminase levels than in alcoholic hepatitis.

2x ULN = If the ALP exceeds this upper limit of normal (ULN) threshold in the setting of a culprit medication (eg, erythromycin, estrogen, rifampin, amoxicillin, chlorpromazine), then drug-induced cholestasis is likely.

Spiegel BMR, Karsan HA.
*Acing the Hepatology Questions on the GI Board
Exam: The Ultimate Crunch-Time Resource (pp 215-220)*
© 2012 SLACK Incorporated

Similarly, if the ALP:AST ratio exceeds 2, then this is a supportive criterion for canalicular ("bland")-type cholestasis.

2.5 mg/dL = If the ascitic fluid total protein exceeds this level with a SAAG ≥1.1, then cardiac ascites, Budd-Chiari syndrome, or myxedema from hypothyroidism is in the differential diagnosis.

3 cm = Maximum allowable size for multifocal hepatocellular carcinoma (HCC) lesions in order to remain eligible for liver transplantation, assuming there are no more than 3 total lesions and there is no metastatic disease and no vascular invasion (Milan criterion—see "5 cm" threshold for an additional Milan criterion).

3x ULN = If ALT is above this threshold in the setting of acute pancreatitis, then the positive predictive value for a gallstone etiology is 95%.

3.4 mg/dL = If serum creatinine exceeds this level in the setting of acetaminophen-induced acute liver failure, then it portends a poor prognosis if INR >6.5 and there is grade 3 or 4 encephalopathy (per King's College criteria).

3.9 mcg/L = An AFP of 3.9 mcg/L on day 1 after peak ALT can be used to predict survival in acetaminophen-induced liver failure with a sensitivity of 100%, a specificity of 74%, a positive predictive value of 45%, and a negative predictive value of 100%.

4 weeks = Undetectable hepatitis C virus (HCV) RNA at this treatment milestone indicates a rapid virologic response (RVR). The likelihood of treatment success with sustained virologic response (SVR) is 90% when an RVR is achieved.

5 = If the ratio of AST:ALP exceeds this threshold in the setting of a culprit medication, then it suggests a hepatocellular form of drug-induced liver injury.

5 cm = Maximum allowable size for a solitary HCC lesion in order to remain eligible for liver transplantation, provided there is no vascular invasion and no metastatic disease (Milan criterion).

5% = Brain uptake of technetium macroaggregated albumin (TcMAA) exceeding this amount indicates intrapulmonary shunting and supports a diagnosis of hepatopulmonary syndrome (HPS) assuming hypoxemia (PaO_2 <70 mm Hg) and an A-a gradient >20 mm Hg.

5x ULN = If the AST exceeds this threshold in autoimmune hepatitis (AIH), <u>and</u> the gamma globulin concurrently exceeds >2x the ULN, then consider starting medical therapy. Of course, there are other indications to begin treatment for AIH—see other thresholds later in this list.

6 = Minimum possible Model for End-Stage Liver Disease (MELD) score.

6 months = If a patient with resectable HCC is unlikely to receive an orthotopic liver transplantation (OLT) for at least this amount of time, then initiation of locoregional bridge therapy with radiofrequency ablation (RFA) or transarterial chemoembolization (TACE) is reasonable while awaiting OLT.

6.5 = If INR exceeds this level in the setting of acetaminophen-induced acute liver failure in conjunction with creatinine >3.4 and grade 3 or 4 encephalopathy, then it portends a poor prognosis (per King's College criteria).

6 to 12 cm = Normal span of the liver by percussion.

7.3 = If arterial pH falls below this value after fluid resuscitation in the setting of acetaminophen-induced acute liver failure, then it portends a poor prognosis (per King's College criteria).

7.5 g = If more than this amount of acetaminophen is consumed at once, then acetaminophen can be hepatotoxic even to a patient without pre-existing liver disease.

10 mmol/L = The goal of diuretic therapy is to induce natriuresis, defined by a spot urine sodium exceeding this threshold.

10 cm = If an echinococcal liver cyst exceeds this size, then it likely requires surgery for definitive therapy due to high risk of rupture.

10x ULN = If the AST exceeds this threshold in AIH, then consider starting medical therapy regardless of the gamma globulin level.

12 g = Quantity of alcohol in a standard alcoholic drink in the United States.

12 mm Hg = If the hepatic venous pressure gradient (HVPG) exceeds this value, then variceal formation is enhanced. Goal of beta-blocker therapy is to reduce the pressure to beneath this threshold.

12 weeks = A 2-log drop or more in HCV RNA at this treatment milestone indicates an early virologic response, or EVR. When an EVR is achieved, the likelihood of achieving an SVR is 66% in genotype 1 HCV.

13 to 15 mg/kg/day = Target range for therapeutic dosing of ursodeoxycholic acid for management of primary biliary cirrhosis (PBC) and intrahepatic cholestasis of pregnancy (ICP).

15 = Usual minimal MELD listing score for liver transplantation.

15 mm Hg = Pulmonary capillary wedge pressure must be below this threshold in order to diagnose portopulmonary hypertension, assuming the mean pulmonary artery pressure (MPAP) is above 25 mm Hg and the pulmonary vascular resistance (PVR) is above 240 dynes/s/cm^{-5}.

20 mg/dL = Ceruloplasmin levels below this value are sensitive (but not specific) for Wilson disease.

20 mm Hg = A-a gradient must exceed this threshold in order to diagnose HPS, assuming there is hypoxemia with PaO_2 <70 mm Hg.

20 mm Hg = Goal of treatment in acute liver failure complicated by elevated intracranial pressure is to drop intracranial pressure below this threshold.

22 = Automatic MELD score initially assigned by the United Network of Organ Sharing (UNOS) for a patient with HCC that fits Milan criteria, regardless of other MELD parameters.

24 weeks = Usual treatment course for genotype 2 or 3 HCV.

25 = Body mass index (BMI) at or above this threshold defines "overweight."

25 mm Hg = MPAP must be above this threshold in order to diagnose portopulmonary hypertension, assuming the PVR is above 240 dynes/s/cm^{-5} and the pulmonary capillary wedge pressure is less than 15 mm Hg.

30 = BMI at or above this threshold defines "obesity."

32 = If the Maddrey discriminant function score (4.6 x Δ prothrombin time + total bilirubin) is above this value in acute alcoholic hepatitis, then consider starting steroids or pentoxiphylline.

34 weeks = Weeks of gestation at which an HBeAg-positive mother with elevated hepatitis B virus (HBV) DNA level should begin oral anti-HBV therapy to minimize vertical transmission of HBV to the newborn.

35 mm Hg = Maximum MPAP often considered acceptable for liver transplantation in the setting of portopulmonary hypertension.

40 = BMI at or above this threshold defines "morbid obesity."

40 = Maximum possible MELD score.

40 μmol/L = When the serum concentration of bile acids exceeds this value in pregnancy, the risk of developing complications from ICP increases significantly.

40% = Brain uptake of TcMAA exceeding this amount is a poor prognostic indicator in HPS indicating a high level of shunting and is a contraindication to liver transplantation.

48 weeks = Usual treatment course for genotype 1 HCV.

50 = Goal in hereditary hemochromatosis is to drive ferritin below this level.

50 mm Hg = PaO$_2$ below this threshold is a poor prognostic indicator in HPS and a contraindication to liver transplantation.

50 to 60 mm Hg = Goal in acute liver failure is to keep cerebral perfusion pressure (CPP) above this threshold (CPP = mean arterial pressure – intracranial pressure).

70 mm Hg = PaO$_2$ must fall below this threshold in order to diagnose HPS, assuming the A-a gradient is above 20 mm Hg.

72 weeks = Length of therapy recommended for hepatitis C genotype 1 patients who are "slow responders"—not the traditional 48 weeks.

78 mEq/L = Goal of diuretic therapy in cirrhotic ascites is to achieve at least this amount of sodium excretion over a 24-hour urine collection. Because a 24-hour collection is often difficult to obtain, most use a spot urine to estimate what a 24-hour collection might have yielded. A urine sodium:potassium ratio >1.0 predicts ≥78 mEq/L of sodium excretion in a 24-hour collection.

88 = If platelet count is below this value in cirrhosis, then the risk of underlying varices increases substantially.

100 mcg/24 hours = Urinary copper excretion above this level is found in almost all symptomatic patients with Wilson disease.

240 dynes/s/cm^{-5} = PVR must exceed this threshold in order to diagnose portopulmonary hypertension, assuming the pulmonary capillary wedge pressure is below 15 mm Hg and the MPAP is >25 mm Hg.

250 = If the PMN count in ascites exceeds this value in cirrhosis, then the patient likely has spontaneous bacterial peritonitis (SBP).

250 mcg/g = Hepatic copper concentration above this level occurs in Wilson disease.

500 mL = Physiologically, this is the maximum amount of ascites that can be absorbed from the peritoneum in 1 day.

1000 ng/mL = A patient under 40 years old with hemochromatosis who has a ferritin value less than 1000 ng/mL is unlikely to have underlying cirrhosis, and liver biopsy can often be avoided.

5700 = 6-methylmercaptopurine levels above 5700 are associated with increased risk of hepatotoxicity when using azathioprine or 6-mercaptopurine.

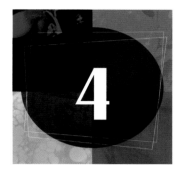

"CRUNCH-TIME" SELF-TEST
TIME TO GET YOUR GAME ON

This is a rapid-fire "crunch-time" self-test. The questions in this test are loosely based on the "Here's the Point!" bullet points from the vignettes. These points represent the distilled essence of potential Board vignettes, so know them well. Some of the questions, however, are stand-alone questions that do not have a corresponding vignette in the book. They are included to test overall background knowledge as opposed to book memorization.

As you read each one-liner, write the answer on the corresponding blank line. Really ... just actively write it right there on the page. Many of the questions ask you to make a diagnosis based on the information given. Although Board questions often ask about much more than the mere diagnosis, you will need to know the diagnosis in order to know what to do next. So, these questions are a bottom-line test of your basic diagnostic capabilities for the "tough stuff" that might show up on the exam.

Very few of these questions are true "gimmies." But if you have carefully studied the vignettes up to this point, then this should be a relative snap—and should reaffirm that you are well on your way to acing the tough stuff. Once you are done, check the answer key on page 237 and score yourself.

Try not to cheat too much as you score your test. If you cheat your way through this, then you won't really know how you did and you won't be able to interpret your score according to the guide on page 243. Once you have finished scoring your test, look up the corresponding vignettes for each of the items you got wrong, and then study those vignettes carefully to fill in your knowledge gaps.

Spiegel BMR, Karsan HA.
Acing the Hepatology Questions on the GI Board Exam: The Ultimate Crunch-Time Resource (pp 221-236)
© 2012 SLACK Incorporated

Question 1. Arrhythmias + Liver test abnormalities + Phospholipid-laden lysosomal lamellar bodies in hepatocytes.

▶ Diagnosis_____

Question 2. Health freak develops elevated liver tests and has lipid-filled stellate cells on liver biopsy.

▶ Diagnosis_____

Question 3. Liver lesion that yields "anchovy paste" upon aspiration.

▶ Diagnosis_____

Question 4. Isolated fundic varices in the setting of chronic pancreatitis.

▶ Diagnosis_____

Question 5. Upper respiratory tract infection + Cholestasis.

▶ Diagnosis_____

Question 6. Acute liver failure upon withdrawal of steroids in polyarteritis nodosa.

▶ Diagnosis_____

Question 7. Hepatitis C + Treatment + Infraumbilical necrotic lesion.

▶ Diagnosis_____

Question 8. Hepatitis C + Lower extremity rash + Positive rheumatoid factor + Renal disease.

▶ Diagnosis_____

Question 9. Hepatitis C + Treatment + Confluent erythematous rash or pruritus.

▶ Diagnosis_____

Question 10. ALT and AST in 1000+ range with ALT:LDH ratio above 1.5 with fever, malaise, and no abdominal pain.

▶ Diagnosis #1_____

▶ Diagnosis #2_____

Question 11. Unexplained elevated aminotransferases + Chronic IBS symptoms.
▶ Diagnosis_____

Question 12. Crohn's disease + Scaling rash + Low ALP.
▶ Diagnosis_____

Question 13. Liver failure during a marathon.
▶ Diagnosis_____

Question 14. Acute hepatitis + Hemolytic anemia + Low ALP.
▶ Diagnosis_____

Question 15. Hepatitis C + Bullae and vesicles on sun-exposed skin.
▶ Diagnosis_____

Question 16. Hepatic bruit + Recent abdominal stab wound.
▶ Diagnosis_____

Question 17. Most likely cause of pancreatitis when the ALT is markedly elevated.
▶ Diagnosis_____

Question 18. Florid duct lesion + Mallory bodies.
▶ Diagnosis_____

Question 19. Hepatitis + Hypouricemia + Mallory bodies.
▶ Diagnosis_____

Question 20. Liver problems with risus sardonicus and micrographia.
▶ Diagnosis_____

Question 21. Metabolic syndrome + Low AST:ALT ratio + Mallory bodies.
▶ Diagnosis_____

Question 22. Mastalgia with ascites treatment.

▶ Diagnosis_____

Question 23. Premature gray hair + Dyspepsia + Macrocytosis + Low ALP.

▶ Diagnosis_____

Question 24. Acute liver failure with persistent hypotension and no evidence of sepsis, neurologic, or cardiogenic shock.

▶ Diagnosis_____

Question 25. Gastroparesis + Cholestasis.

▶ Diagnosis_____

Question 26. Caudate lobe hypertrophy.

▶ Diagnosis_____

Question 27. ≥2-log drop in HCV RNA but detectable virus at week 12; undetectable RNA at week 24.

▶ Diagnosis_____

Question 28. Hepatic abscess in traveler with elevation of right hemidiaphragm with adhesions obliterating the costophrenic angle.

▶ Diagnosis_____

Question 29. Dermatographism + Hepatomegaly + Pruritus + Flushing + Elevated ALP.

▶ Diagnosis_____

Question 30. New-onset continuous periumbilical humming sound in a patient with cirrhosis with recent improvement of ascites.

▶ Diagnosis_____

Question 31. Acute liver failure after eating some botanicals on a nature walk in Ireland.

▶ Diagnosis_____

Question 32. Hepatic bruit + Sudden high AST:ALT ratio + History of recurrent pancreatitis.

▶ Diagnosis_____

Question 33. Sheepherder with liver cyst with "eggshell calcifications" and septations.

▶ Diagnosis_____

Question 34. ANA positive + SMA positive + AMA negative + Elevated ALP.

▶ Diagnosis_____

Question 35. High SAAG, high protein ascites + Fatigue + Constipation + Low ALP.

▶ Diagnosis_____

Question 36. Polycythemia vera + Hepatomegaly.

▶ Diagnosis_____

Question 37. Liver mass with central stellate scar without growth on serial imaging.

▶ Diagnosis_____

Question 38. Anabolic steroids + Subcapsular liver mass with arterial enhancement.

▶ Diagnosis_____

Question 39. "Stepwise" fever + Temperature-pulse dissociation + "Rose spots" + Hepatitis.

▶ Diagnosis_____

Question 40. Undetectable HCV RNA by week 4.

▶ Diagnosis_____

Question 41. Undetectable HCV RNA by week 12.

▶ Diagnosis_____

Question 42. Undetectable HCV RNA 6 months after completion of treatment course.

▸ Diagnosis_____

Question 43. Sheepherder develops biliary obstruction and hepatomegaly, and has "tortuous tracks" in liver on CT.

▸ Diagnosis_____

Question 44. IBD patient gets painful hepatomegaly, ascites, and a high bilirubin after starting azathioprine.

▸ Diagnosis_____

Question 45. Spider web collaterals on hepatic venography.

▸ Diagnosis_____

Question 46. Chronically unexplained elevation of aminotransferases + Vesicular elbow rash + Iron deficiency anemia.

▸ Diagnosis_____

Question 47. Hepatic bruit + Long-standing hemochromatosis + New-onset encephalopathy.

▸ Diagnosis_____

Question 48. A bodybuilder develops a rare liver tumor (not hepatocellular carcinoma).

▸ Diagnosis_____

Question 49. Cause of biliary ductal fibrosis and gallstones in someone who eats lots of undercooked seafood.

▸ Diagnosis_____

Question 50. Worms in the biliary tree after eating contaminated freshwater plants.

▸ Diagnosis_____

Question 51. Lots and lots of biliary and intrahepatic pigment stones, but a normal gallbladder.

▸ Diagnosis_____

Question 52. Anicteric acute liver failure with fever, leukopenia, and abnormal chest X-ray.
▶ Diagnosis_____

Question 53. Genetic polymorphisms of this gene explain variations in HCV treatment success among patients with different ancestry.
▶ Gene_____

Question 54. "Owl's eye" intranuclear hepatocyte inclusions.
▶ Diagnosis_____

Question 55. Sexually active woman with fever, right upper quadrant pain, abnormal aminotransferase with enhancement of the anterior liver capsule on arterial phase of the CT undergoes laparoscopy notable for "violin string" perihepatic adhesions.
▶ Diagnosis_____

Question 56. Acute liver failure in HBV carrier with active drug abuse with the following serologies: hepatitis B core IgM negative, hepatitis B DNA 75 IU/mL, hepatitis A IgG positive, HCV RNA negative.
▶ Diagnosis_____

Question 57. Patient with a history of pancreatitis that responded to a course of tapering medication now presents with elevated ALP and GGT. MRCP reveals a "chain of lakes" appearance in the biliary tree.
▶ Diagnosis_____

Question 58. Cough + Liver cyst with septations.
▶ Diagnosis_____

Question 59. Most heavily weighted variable in the MELD scoring system.
▶ Variable_____

Question 60. Circle the clinical consequences of hereditary hemochromatosis that can improve with successful phlebotomy:
    Arthropathy
    Hypogonadism
    Decompensated cirrhosis
    Cutaneous hyperpigmentation
    Diabetes

Question 61. Liver mass with calcifications and a central scar in the absence of cirrhosis.

▶ Diagnosis_____

Question 62. Undetectable HCV RNA at completion of therapy.

▶ Diagnosis_____

Question 63. Portal vein granuloma + Portal hypertension + Absence of other stigmata of chronic liver disease + Eosinophilia.

▶ Diagnosis_____

Question 64. Liver disease + Parkinsonian tremor + Fanconi syndrome.

▶ Diagnosis_____

Question 65. Sunflower cataracts.

▶ Diagnosis_____

Question 66. Acute hepatitis + Hyperthermia + Bruxism + Young adult.

▶ Diagnosis_____

Question 67. Anaphylaxis after a liver cyst filled with "sand" ruptures.

▶ Diagnosis_____

Question 68. Unexplained elevated aminotransferases + Short statured + Osteopenia + Infertility + Bloating.

▶ Diagnosis_____

Question 69. Proximal muscle weakness + 10-fold elevations of AST and ALT + Normal total bilirubin, INR, and ALP.

▶ Diagnosis_____

Question 70. Patient with precirrhotic PBC becomes tired and constipated.

▶ Diagnosis_____

Question 71. Patient with PSC develops easy bruisability and elevated INR after starting antibiotic treatment for cholangitis.

▸ Diagnosis_____

Question 72. Patient with PBC develops progressive night blindness.

▸ Diagnosis_____

Question 73. Patient with PBC develops problems with balance and gait in the absence of hepatic encephalopathy.

▸ Diagnosis_____

Question 74. Pregnant woman with fatigue, polyuria, palmar erythema, spider angiomas, and small esophageal varices.

▸ Most common diagnosis_____

Question 75. Pregnant woman with cirrhosis presenting with a left upper quadrant discomfort and bruit.

▸ Diagnosis_____

Question 76. A patient receives a new medication for her seizure disorder. A month later she is found to have elevated liver tests. A subsequent liver biopsy reveals microvesicular steatosis.

▸ Diagnosis_____

Question 77. Hyperpigmentation + Arthropathy + High ferritin + Abnormal echocardiogram.

▸ Diagnosis_____

Questions 78 to 80. Patient comes from Puerto Rico with diarrhea, malabsorption, and flat villi on endoscopy. He develops elevated AST and ALT after beginning therapy for his condition. (Name the condition, medication, and type of hepatotoxicity with the medication.)

▸ 78. Diagnosis_____

▸ 79. Medication_____

▸ 80. Hepatotoxicity_____

Question 81. Most favorable IL28B polymorphism genotype.

▶ Genotype_____

Question 82. Obese patient with diabetes has a 5-cm irregular, hypoechoic lesion in the right hepatic lobe. Follow-up CT reveals a hypodense, sharply demarcated mass. The contour and architecture are otherwise not distorted, with vascular structures passing through the mass normally.

▶ Diagnosis_____

Question 83. Patient with essential thrombocytosis has isolated, elevated ALP. CT reveals multiple hypodense nodules. Biopsy reveals regenerative nodules clustered around portal triads without fibrosis between the nodules.

▶ Diagnosis_____

Question 84. Asian patient with Crohn's disease starts infliximab and develops acute liver failure. What underlying infection may have done this?

▶ Diagnosis_____

Question 85. HBeAg-positive patient with high HBV viral load is pregnant at week 34. What can be done to minimize vertical transmission to the newborn?

▶ Treatment_____

Questions 86 to 87. Patient eats an *Amanita* mushroom and develops acute liver failure. Name 2 specific therapies for this particular form of liver failure.

▶ 86. Therapy #1_____

▶ 87. Therapy #2_____

Question 88. HBV genotype that is most prevalent among African-Americans.

▶ Genotype_____

Question 89. HBV genotype with best response to interferon therapy.

▶ Genotype_____

Questions 90 to 91. Two most prevalent HBV genotypes among Asian patients.

▶ 90. Genotype_____

▶ 91. Genotype_____

Question 92. HBV genotype that is most prevalent among patients from Eastern Europe.

▶ Genotype_____

Question 93. Traveler to Indian subcontinent develops acute hepatitis despite appropriate pre-travel vaccinations.

▶ Diagnosis_____

Question 94. Pregnant woman develops severe nausea, vomiting, and fatigue at 8 weeks' gestation. Labs include elevated AST, ALT, and mildly elevated bilirubin. There are no ill contacts. Liver biopsy is normal.

▶ Diagnosis_____

Question 95. Most common cause of jaundice in pregnancy.

▶ Diagnosis_____

Question 96. Second leading cause of jaundice in pregnancy.

▶ Diagnosis_____

Question 97. Fever and cutaneous skin eruptions after starting therapy for Wilson disease.

▶ Diagnosis_____

Question 98. People of Chilean descent are especially at risk for developing this liver complication of pregnancy.

▶ Diagnosis_____

Question 99. Pregnant woman in third trimester develops pruritus, subclinical steatorrhea, and vitamin K deficiency.

▶ Diagnosis_____

Question 100. Liver disease of pregnancy resulting from impairment of intramitochondrial fatty acid oxidation from a mutation causing long-chain 3-hydroxyacyl-coenyzme A dehydrogenase (LCHAD) deficiency.

▶ Diagnosis_____

Question 101. Late third trimester pregnancy is complicated by elevated AST, ALT, total bilirubin, creatinine, and INR, along with mental status changes and hypoglycemia.

▸ Diagnosis_____

Question 102. Woman with HELLP syndrome develops severe, acute abdominal pain and hypotension while awaiting emergency C-section.

▸ Diagnosis_____

Question 103. Massive liver cysts + Intracranial aneurysm.

▸ Diagnosis_____

Question 104. Most common malignancy to develop de novo after liver transplantation.

▸ Diagnosis_____

Question 105. Patient with autosomal dominant polycystic kidney disease develops lower abdominal pain and fever and has rebound tenderness on exam.

▸ Diagnosis_____

Question 106. Cirrhosis + Loud P2 + Tricuspid regurgitation + Increased edema.

▸ Diagnosis_____

Question 107. Liver disease + Hypoxemia + Intrapulmonary vasodilation.

▸ Diagnosis_____

Question 108. Liver disease + Hypoxemia + >5% brain uptake of technetium macroaggregated albumin.

▸ Diagnosis_____

Question 109. Patient has a 2-cm left lobe amebic liver abscess.

▸ Treatment_____

Question 110. A 50-year-old patient with cirrhosis with a small, 2-cm HCC. Labs: albumin = 3.5, INR = 1.0, total bilirubin = 1.9, creatinine = 1.0, platelets = 102, AFP = 40.

▶ Best treatment_____

Question 111. DIC + Giant hemangioma.

▶ Diagnosis_____

Question 112. Third-trimester pregnancy is complicated by elevated AST, ALT, total bilirubin, and LDH, along with microangiopathic hemolytic anemia.

▶ Diagnosis_____

Question 113. Patient with cirrhosis with platypnea and orthodeoxia.

▶ Diagnosis_____

Question 114. AIDS + Elevated ALP and GGT + *Bartonella* infection.

▶ Diagnosis_____

Question 115. Patient with CREST syndrome has a high GGT level + Steatorrhea.

▶ Diagnosis_____

Question 116. Patient with acute diverticulitis develops right upper quadrant pain and persistent fever with this nonmalignant liver abnormality on CT.

▶ Diagnosis_____

Question 117. Third-trimester pregnancy is complicated by liver trouble. Biopsy reveals periportal hemorrhage, fibrin deposition in the sinusoids, and focal necrosis.

▶ Diagnosis_____

Question 118. Cause of gram-negative septic shock in Gulf Coast fisherman with cirrhosis and previous leg laceration.

▶ Diagnosis_____

Question 119. Recurrence rate of Wilson disease after liver transplantation.

▶ Recurrence rate_____

Question 120. 35-year-old man with PSC and 1-cm gallbladder polyp.

▶ Recommendation_____

Question 121. Recurrence rate of alpha-1 antitrypsin deficiency (A1AT) after liver transplantation.

▶ Recurrence rate_____

Question 122. Most common phenotype of A1AT.

▶ Phenotype_____

Question 123. Most common A1AT phenotype in patients with A1AT-induced chronic obstructive pulmonary disease.

▶ Phenotype_____

Question 124. Most common A1AT phenotype in patients with A1AT-induced cirrhosis.

▶ Phenotype_____

Question 125. This A1AT phenotype serves an intermediate role with other cofactors that can lead to cirrhosis.

▶ Phenotype_____

Question 126. Most common cause of inherited indirect hyperbilirubinemia that could potentially lead to an artificially high MELD score:

▶ Diagnosis_____

Question 127. Currently the most common indication for liver transplantation in the United States.

▶ Diagnosis_____

Question 128. Based on prognostic models, this will be the most common indication for liver transplantation in the United States 40 years from now.

▶ Diagnosis_____

Question 129. Hepatitis C is an independent risk factor for diabetes mellitus after liver transplantation. (Circle correct answer.)

    True

    False

Question 130. This hepatitis C genotype is associated with NAFLD, which can improve with therapy.

▸ Genotype_____

Question 131. This hepatitis C genotype is highly prevalent in Egypt.

▸ Genotype_____

Question 132. This hepatitis C genotype is highly prevalent in South Africa.

▸ Genotype_____

Question 133. This hepatitis C genotype is highly prevalent in Southeast Asia.

▸ Genotype_____

Questions 134 and 135. These questions concern DAAs and HCV genotype 1 subtype comparisons to one another.

134. Which subtype of HCV genotype 1 is more commonly found in North America and has increased resistance to NS3/4a protease inhibitors?

▸ Subtype_____

135. Which subtype of HCV genotype 1 is more commonly found in Europe and has a decreased resistance to the NS3/4a protease inhibitors?

▸ Subtype_____

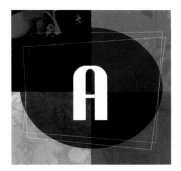

APPENDIX A
ANSWERS TO "CRUNCH-TIME" SELF-TEST

1. Amiodarone hepatotoxicity
2. Hypervitaminosis A
3. Amebic liver abscess
4. Splenic vein thrombosis
5. Cholestasis from trimethoprim-sulfamethoxazole or amoxicillin-clavulanate
6. Acute hepatitis B during immune reconstitution
7. Interferon-induced skin necrosis at injection site
8. Mixed cryoglobulinemia
9. Ribavirin-induced skin rash
10. 1. Acute viral hepatitis 2. Autoimmune hepatitis
11. Celiac sprue
12. Zinc deficiency
13. Acute liver failure from exertional heat stroke
14. Wilson disease
15. Porphyria cutanea tarda
16. Traumatic arteriovenous fistula
17. Gallstones
18. Primary biliary cirrhosis
19. Wilson disease
20. Wilson disease

Spiegel BMR, Karsan HA.
Acing the Hepatology Questions on the GI Board
Exam: The Ultimate Crunch-Time Resource (pp 237-242)
© 2012 SLACK Incorporated

21. Nonalcoholic fatty liver disease
22. Spironolactone-induced gynecomastia
23. Pernicious anemia
24. Adrenal insufficiency
25. Erythromycin-induced cholestasis
26. Budd-Chiari syndrome
27. Partial early virologic response or slow responder
28. Amebic liver abscess
29. Systemic mastocytosis with liver infiltration
30. Cruveilhier-Baumgarten murmur from recanalized umbilical vein
31. *Amanita* mushroom poisoning
32. Alcoholic hepatitis
33. Echinococcosis
34. Autoimmune cholangiopathy
35. Hypothyroidism
36. Budd-Chiari syndrome
37. Focal nodular hyperplasia
38. Hepatic adenoma
39. *Salmonella typhi* hepatitis
40. Rapid virologic response
41. Complete early virologic response
42. Sustained virologic response
43. Fascioliasis
44. Sinusoidal obstruction syndrome (aka veno-occlusive disease)
45. Budd-Chiari syndrome
46. Celiac sprue (with dermatitis herpetiformis)
47. Hepatocellular carcinoma
48. Hepatic angiosarcoma
49. *Clonorchis sinensis*
50. *Fasciola hepatica*
51. Recurrent pyogenic cholangitis
52. Acute herpes hepatitis
53. IL-28B
54. CMV hepatitis
55. Fitz-Hugh–Curtis syndrome

56. Hepatitis D (delta) virus superinfection
57. Autoimmune (IgG4-associated) cholangitis
58. Echinococcal (hydatid) cyst
59. INR
60. Cutaneous hyperpigmentation and diabetes
61. Fibrolamellar hepatocellular carcinoma
62. End of treatment response
63. Schistosomiasis
64. Wilson disease (yes, again)
65. Wilson disease (know it)
66. Ecstasy overdose
67. Echinococcal (hydatid) cyst
68. Celiac sprue
69. Myositis
70. Autoimmune-related hypothyroidism
71. Vitamin K deficiency
72. Vitamin A deficiency
73. Vitamin E deficiency
74. Normal pregnancy
75. Splenic artery aneurysm
76. Valproic acid hepatotoxicity
77. Hemochromatosis
78. Condition: tropical sprue
79. Medication: tetracycline
80. Side effect: microvesicular steatosis
81. CC
82. Focal fatty infiltration (not a tumor)
83. Nodular regenerative hyperplasia
84. Hepatitis B
85. Start oral antiviral in mom; newborn receives HBIG and HBV vaccination
86. Therapy #1: Penicillin G
87. Therapy #2: Milk thistle (silymarin)
88. Genotype A
89. Genotype A
90. Genotype B or C

91. Genotype C or B
92. Genotype D
93. Hepatitis E
94. Hyperemesis gravidarum
95. Viral hepatitis
96. Intrahepatic cholestasis of pregnancy
97. D-Penicillamine acute hypersensitivity reaction
98. Intrahepatic cholestasis of pregnancy
99. Intrahepatic cholestasis of pregnancy
100. Acute fatty liver of pregnancy
101. Acute fatty liver of pregnancy
102. Subcapsular hematoma or rupture
103. Autosomal dominant polycystic kidney disease
104. Squamous cell skin cancer
105. Acute diverticulitis
106. Portopulmonary hypertension
107. Hepatopulmonary syndrome
108. Hepatopulmonary syndrome
109. Surgical drainage procedure
110. Refer for transplant
111. Kasabach-Merritt syndrome
112. HELLP syndrome
113. Hepatopulmonary syndrome
114. Peliosis hepatis
115. May be PBC
116. Pyogenic liver abscess
117. HELLP syndrome
118. *Vibrio vulnificus*
119. 0% (cured)
120. Cholecystectomy
121. 0% (cured)
122. MM
123. ZZ
124. ZZ
125. MZ

126. Gilbert's syndrome

127. Hepatitis C

128. NAFLD or NASH

129. True

130. Genotype 3

131. Genotype 4

132. Genotype 5

133. Genotype 6 (Genotypes 7, 8, 9, 10, and 11 also found in Southeast Asia)

134. Genotype 1a

135. Genotype 1b

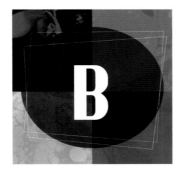

APPENDIX B
"CRUNCH-TIME" SELF-TEST
SCORING GUIDE

135 correct:	You cheated.
130–134:	You still cheated.
125–129:	Impossible to believe.
120–124:	Either you cheated, or you're a monster diagnostician ready to crush the Boards.
115–119:	Assuming you didn't cheat, that was a crazy good performance.
110–114:	Outstanding performance—easily more than a standard deviation above the mean.
105–109:	Pretty darn tremendous.
100–104:	Highly respectable—well above average for this level of difficulty.
95–109:	Good work—you're definitely ahead of the curve.
90–94:	You're doing fine—a good effort.
85–89:	Don't despair—these are hard, and you hung in well.
80–84:	Not terrible, but you need to start fine-tuning the rough spots.
75–79:	Could be better.
70–74:	Look in the mirror. Then say, "I know I can do better. Let's kick this up a notch."
65–69:	You're in the 50% range now—mediocre.
60–64:	Not good enough—below average.
55–59:	These are tough, but you're below the curve.
50–54:	Inadequate knowledge base. You're in jeopardy of not passing the exam.
<50:	Wait a while before taking the exam. You've got a ways to go.

Spiegel BMR, Karsan HA.
Acing the Hepatology Questions on the GI Board
Exam: The Ultimate Crunch-Time Resource (pp 243-244)
© 2012 SLACK Incorporated

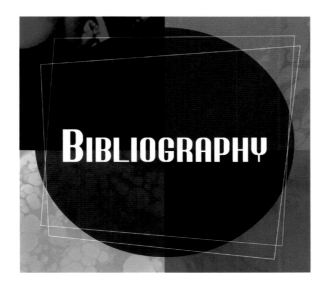

BIBLIOGRAPHY

Adams LA, Lymp JF, St Sauver J, et al. The natural history of nonalcoholic fatty liver disease: a population-based cohort study. *Gastroenterology.* 2005;129:113-121.

Aggarwal R, Naik S. Epidemiology of hepatitis E: current status. *J Gastroenterol Hepatol.* 2009;24:1484-1493.

Anand AC, Nightingale P, Neuberger JM. Early indicators of prognosis in fulminant hepatic failure: an assessment of the King's criteria. *J Hepatol.* 1997;26:62-68.

Andreu V, Mas A, Bruguera M, et al. Ecstasy: a common cause of severe acute hepatotoxicity. *J Hepatol.* 1998;29:394-397.

Angulo P, Dickson ER, Therneau TM, et al. Comparison of three doses of ursodeoxycholic acid in the treatment of primary biliary cirrhosis: a randomized trial. *J Hepatol.* 1999;30:830-835.

Arguedas MR, Abrams GA, Krowka MJ, Fallon MB. Prospective evaluation of outcomes and predictors of mortality in patients with hepatopulmonary syndrome undergoing liver transplantation. *Hepatology.* 2003;37:192-197.

Bacon BR. Hemochromatosis: diagnosis and management. *Gastroenterology.* 2001;120:718-725.

Bacon BR, Gordon SC, Lawitz E, et al. Boceprevir for previously treated chronic HCV genotype 1 infection. *N Engl J Med.* 2011;364:1207-1217.

Bacq Y, Zarka O, Brechot JF, et al. Liver function tests in normal pregnancy: a prospective study of 103 pregnant women and 103 matched controls. *Hepatology.* 1996;23:1030-1034.

Bader T. The myth of statin-induced hepatotoxicity. *Am J Gastroenterol.* 2010;105:978-980.

Bass NM, Mullen KD, Sanyal A, et al. Rifaximin treatment in hepatic encephalopathy. *N Engl J Med.* 2010;362:1071-1081.

Berger J, Hart J, Millis M, Baker AL. Fulminant hepatic failure from heat stroke requiring liver transplantation. *J Clin Gastroenterol.* 2000;30:429-431.

Bonora E, Targher G, Alberiche M, et al. Homeostasis model assessment closely mirrors the glucose clamp technique in the assessment of insulin sensitivity: studies in subjects with various degrees of glucose tolerance and insulin sensitivity. *Diabetes Care.* 2000;23:57-63.

Bornstein JD, Byrd DE, Trotter JF. Relapsing hepatitis A: a case report and review of the literature. *J Clin Gastroenterol.* 1999;28:355-356.

Boyer TD, Haskal ZJ. The role of transjugular intrahepatic portosystemic shunt (TIPS) in the management of portal hypertension: update 2009. *Hepatology.* 2010;51:306.

Bravi F, Bosetti C, Tavani A, et al. Coffee drinking and hepatocellular carcinoma risk: a meta-analysis. *Hepatology.* 2007;46:430-435.

Broome U, Glaumann H, Lindstom E, et al. Natural history and outcome in 32 Swedish patients with small duct primary sclerosing cholangitis (PSC). *J Hepatol.* 2002;36:586-589.

Broome U, Lofberg R, Veress B, Eriksson LS. Primary sclerosing cholangitis and ulcerative colitis: evidence for increased neoplastic potential. *Hepatology.* 1995;22:1404-1408.

Buckles DC, Lindor KD, Larusso NF, Petrovic LM, Gores GJ. In primary sclerosing cholangitis, gallbladder polyps are frequently malignant. *Am J Gastroenterol.* 2002;97:1138-1142.

Burak K, Angulo P, Pasha TM, Egan K, Petz J, Lindor KD. Incidence and risk factors for cholangiocarcinoma in primary sclerosing cholangitis. *Am J Gastroenterol.* 2004;99:523-526.

Carvalho M, Pontes H, Remiao F, Bastos ML, Carvalho F. Mechanisms underlying the hepatotoxic effects of ecstasy. *Curr Pharm Biotechnol.* 2010;11:476-495.

Cassidy WM, Reynolds TB. Serum lactic dehydrogenase in the differential diagnosis of acute hepatocellular injury. *J Clin Gastroenterol.* 1994;19:118-121.

Chapman R, Fevery J, Kalloo A, et al. Diagnosis and management of primary sclerosing cholangitis. *Hepatology.* 2010;51:660-678.

Claessen MM, Vleggaar FP, Tytgat KM, Siersema PD, van Buuren HR. High lifetime risk of cancer in primary sclerosing cholangitis. *J Hepatol.* 2009;50:158-164.

Colina F, Pinedo F, Solis JA, Moreno D, Nevado M. Nodular regenerative hyperplasia of the liver in early histological stages of primary biliary cirrhosis. *Gastroenterology.* 1992;102:1319-1324.

Colombato L. The role of transjugular intrahepatic portosystemic shunt (TIPS) in the management of portal hypertension. *J Clin Gastroenterol.* 2007;41(suppl 3):S344-S351.

Compston A. Progressive lenticular degeneration: a familial nervous disease associated with cirrhosis of the liver. by S. A. Kinnier Wilson (From the National Hospital, and the Laboratory of the National Hospital, Queen Square, London), *Brain* 1912: 34; 295-509. *Brain* 2009;132:1997-2001.

Conroy M, Sewell L, Miller OF, Ferringer T. Interferon-beta injection site reaction: review of the histology and report of a lupus-like pattern. *J Am Acad Dermatol.* 2008;59:S48-S49.

Corigliano N, Mercantini P, Amodio PM, et al. Hemoperitoneum from a spontaneous rupture of a giant hemangioma of the liver: report of a case. *Surg Today.* 2003;33:459-463.

de Castro F, Bonacini M, Walden JM, Schubert TT. Myxedema ascites. Report of two cases and review of the literature. *J Clin Gastroenterol.* 1991;13:411-414.

Dolapci M, Ersoz S, Kama NA. Hepatic artery aneurysm. *Ann Vasc Surg.* 2003;17:214-216.

Elmberg M, Hultcrantz R, Ekbom A, et al. Cancer risk in patients with hereditary hemochromatosis and in their first-degree relatives. *Gastroenterology.* 2003;125:1733-1741.

El-Newihi HM, Alamy ME, Reynolds TB. Salmonella hepatitis: analysis of 27 cases and comparison with acute viral hepatitis. *Hepatology.* 1996;24:516-519.

El-Serag HB, Davila JA, Petersen NJ, McGlynn KA. The continuing increase in the incidence of hepatocellular carcinoma in the United States: an update. *Ann Intern Med.* 2003;139:817-823.

El-Serag HB, Siegel AB, Davila JA, et al. Treatment and outcomes of treating of hepatocellular carcinoma among Medicare recipients in the United States: a population-based study. *J Hepatol.* 2006;44:158-166.

Elta GH, Sepersky RA, Goldberg MJ, Connors CM, Miller KB, Kaplan MM. Increased incidence of hypothyroidism in primary biliary cirrhosis. *Dig Dis Sci.* 1983;28:971-975.

Esrailian E, Pantangco ER, Kyulo NL, Hu KQ, Runyon BA. Octreotide/Midodrine therapy significantly improves renal function and 30-day survival in patients with type 1 hepatorenal syndrome. *Dig Dis Sci.* 2007;52:742-748.

European Association for the Study of the Liver. EASL Clinical Practice Guidelines: management of cholestatic liver diseases. *J Hepatol.* 2009;51:237-267.

European Association for the Study of the Liver. EASL Clinical Practice Guidelines: management of chronic hepatitis B. *J Hepatol.* 2009;50:227-242.

European Association for the Study of the Liver. EASL Clinical Practice Guidelines for HFE hemochromatosis. *J Hepatol.* 2010;53:3-22.

Euvrard S, Kanitakis J, Claudy A. Skin cancers after organ transplantation. *N Engl J Med.* 2003;348:1681-1691.

Fasano A, Berti I, Gerarduzzi T, et al. Prevalence of celiac disease in at-risk and not-at-risk groups in the United States: a large multicenter study. *Arch Intern Med.* 2003;163:286-292.

Favennec L, Jave Ortiz J, Gargala G, Lopez Chegne N, Ayoub A, Rossignol JF. Double-blind, randomized, placebo-controlled study of nitazoxanide in the treatment of fascioliasis in adults and children from northern Peru. *Aliment Pharmacol Ther.* 2003;17:265-270.

Fevery J, Verslype C, Lai G, Aerts R, Van Steenbergen W. Incidence, diagnosis, and therapy of cholangiocarcinoma in patients with primary sclerosing cholangitis. *Dig Dis Sci.* 2007;52:3123-3135.

Foley WJ, Turcotte JG, Hoskins PA, Brant RL, Ause RG. Intrahepatic arteriovenous fistulas between the hepatic artery and portal vein. *Ann Surg.* 1971;174:849-855.

Ford AC, Chey WD, Talley NJ, Malhotra A, Spiegel BM, Moayyedi P. Yield of diagnostic tests for celiac disease in individuals with symptoms suggestive of irritable bowel syndrome: systematic review and meta-analysis. *Arch Intern Med*. 2009;169:651-658.

Freedman ND, Curto TM, Lindsay KL, Wright EC, Sinha R, Everhart JE; HALT-C Trial Group. Coffee consumption is associated with response to peginterferon and ribavirin therapy in patients with chronic hepatitis C. *Gastroenterology*. 2011;140:1961-1969.

Ge D, Fellay J, Thompson AJ, et al. Genetic variation in IL28B predicts hepatitis C treatment-induced viral clearance. *Nature*. 2009;461:399-401.

Gleisner AL, Munoz A, Brandao A, et al. Survival benefit of liver transplantation and the effect of underlying liver disease. *Surgery*. 2010;147:392-404.

Gordon SC, Reddy KR, Schiff L, Schiff ER. Prolonged intrahepatic cholestasis secondary to acute hepatitis A. *Ann Intern Med*. 1984;101:635-637.

Gordon-Weeks AN, Snaith A, Petrinic T. Systematic review of outcome of downstaging hepatocellular cancer before liver transplantation in patients outside the Milan criteria. *Br J Surg*. 2011;54:645-647.

Guillevin L, Mahr A, Callard P, et al. Hepatitis B virus-associated polyarteritis nodosa: clinical characteristics, outcome, and impact of treatment in 115 patients. *Medicine (Baltimore)*. 2005;84:313-322.

Gumaste VV, Dave PB, Weissman D, Messer J. Lipase/amylase ratio. A new index that distinguishes acute episodes of alcoholic from nonalcoholic acute pancreatitis. *Gastroenterology*. 1991;101:1361-1366.

Hadad E, Ben-Ari Z, Heled Y, Moran DS, Shani Y, Epstein Y. Liver transplantation in exertional heat stroke: a medical dilemma. *Intensive Care Med*. 2004;30:1474-1478.

Hall GW. Kasabach-Merritt syndrome: pathogenesis and management. *Br J Haematol*. 2001;112:851-862.

Hans D, Durosier C, Kanis JA, Johansson H, Schott-Pethelaz AM, Krieg MA. Assessment of the 10-year probability of osteoporotic hip fracture combining clinical risk factors and heel bone ultrasound: the EPISEM prospective cohort of 12,958 elderly women. *J Bone Miner Res*. 2008;23:1045-1051.

Haque R, Huston CD, Hughes M, Houpt E, Petri WA Jr. Amebiasis. *N Engl J Med*. 2003;348:1565-1573.

Harrison PM, Keays R, Bray GP, Alexander GJ, Williams R. Improved outcome of paracetamol-induced fulminant hepatic failure by late administration of acetylcysteine. *Lancet*. 1990;335:1572-1573.

Harry R, Auzinger G, Wendon J. The clinical importance of adrenal insufficiency in acute hepatic dysfunction. *Hepatology*. 2002;36:395-402.

Hashimoto E, Taniai M, Kaneda H, et al. Comparison of hepatocellular carcinoma patients with alcoholic liver disease and nonalcoholic steatohepatitis. *Alcohol Clin Exp Res*. 2004;28:164S-168S.

Hashimoto E, Yatsuji S, Tobari M, et al. Hepatocellular carcinoma in patients with nonalcoholic steatohepatitis. *J Gastroenterol*. 2009;44(suppl 19):89-95.

Hay JE. Liver disease in pregnancy. *Hepatology*. 2008;47:1067-1076.

Hazin R, Abu-Rajab Tamimi TI, Abuzetun JY, Zein NN. Recognizing and treating cutaneous signs of liver disease. *Cleve Clin J Med*. 2009;76:599-606.

McHutchinson JG, Everson GT, Gordon SC, et al. Telaprevir with peginterferon and ribavirin for chronic HCV genotype 1 infection. *N Engl J Med*. 2009;360:1827-1938.

McHutchinson JG, Manns MP, Muir AJ, et al. Telaprevir for previously treated chronic HCV infection. *N Engl J Med*. 2010;362:1292-1303.

Hennigar GR, Greene WB, Walker EM, de Saussure C. Hemochromatosis caused by excessive vitamin iron intake. *Am J Pathol*. 1979;96:611-624.

Herbert V. Hemochromatosis and vitamin C. *Ann Intern Med*. 1999;131:475-476.

Hillemanns P, Knitza R, Muller-Hocker J. Rupture of splenic artery aneurysm in a pregnant patient with portal hypertension. *Am J Obstet Gynecol*. 1996;174:1665-1666.

Hoefs JC, Morgan TR. Seventy-two weeks of peginterferon and ribavirin for patients with partial early virologic response? *Hepatology*. 2007;46:1671-1674.

Holtmann M, Schreiner O, Kohler H, et al. Veno-occlusive disease (VOD) in Crohn's disease (CD) treated with azathioprine. *Dig Dis Sci*. 2003;48:1503-1505.

Holubek WJ, Kalman S, Hoffman RS. Acetaminophen-induced acute liver failure: results of a United States multicenter, prospective study. *Hepatology*. 2006;43:880; author reply 882.

Ichai P, Roque Afonso AM, Sebagh M, et al. Herpes simplex virus-associated acute liver failure: a difficult diagnosis with a poor prognosis. *Liver Transpl*. 2005;11:1550-1555.

Iwatsuki S, Todo S, Starzl TE. Excisional therapy for benign hepatic lesions. *Surg Gynecol Obstet*. 1990;171:240-246.

Jensen K, Gluud C. The Mallory body: morphological, clinical and experimental studies (Part 1 of a literature survey). *Hepatology*. 1994;20:1061-1077.

Jones AL, Simpson KJ. Review article: mechanisms and management of hepatotoxicity in ecstasy (MDMA) and amphetamine intoxications. *Aliment Pharmacol Ther*. 1999;13:129-133.

Kanwal F, Gralnek IM, Martin P, Dulai GS, Farid M, Spiegel BM. Treatment alternatives for chronic hepatitis B virus infection: a cost-effectiveness analysis. *Ann Intern Med*. 2005;142:821-831.

Karlsen TH, Schrumpf E, Boberg KM. Gallbladder polyps in primary sclerosing cholangitis: not so benign. *Curr Opin Gastroenterol*. 2008;24:395-399.

Karsan HA, Rojter SE, Saab S. Primary prevention of cirrhosis. Public health strategies that can make a difference. *Postgrad Med*. 2004;115:25-30.

Keeffe EB, Dieterich DT, Han SH, et al. A treatment algorithm for the management of chronic hepatitis B virus infection in the United States: 2008 update. *Clin Gastroenterol Hepatol*. 2008;6:1315-1341; quiz 1286.

Khuroo MS. Hepatitis E virus. *Curr Opin Infect Dis*. 2008;21:539-543.

Kim WR, Biggins SW, Kremers WK, et al. Hyponatremia and mortality among patients on the liver-transplant waiting list. *N Engl J Med*. 2008;359:1018-1026.

Knill-Jones RP, Buckle RM, Parsons V, Calne RY, Williams R. Hypercalcemia and increased parathyroid-hormone activity in a primary hepatoma. Studies before and after hepatic transplantation. *N Engl J Med*. 1970;282:704-708.

Kowdley KV, Brandhagen DJ, Gish RG, et al. Survival after liver transplantation in patients with hepatic iron overload: the national hemochromatosis transplant registry. *Gastroenterology*. 2005;129:494-503.

Krowka MJ, Fallon MB, Mulligan DC, Gish RG. Model for end-stage liver disease (MELD) exception for portopulmonary hypertension. *Liver Transpl*. 2006;12:S114-S116.

Krowka MJ, Swanson KL, Frantz RP, McGoon MD, Wiesner RH. Portopulmonary hypertension: results from a 10-year screening algorithm. *Hepatology*. 2006;44:1502-1510.

Larson AM, Polson J, Fontana RJ, et al. Acetaminophen-induced acute liver failure: results of a United States multicenter, prospective study. *Hepatology*. 2005;42:1364-1372.

Larsson SC, Wolk A. Coffee consumption and risk of liver cancer: a meta-analysis. *Gastroenterology*. 2007;132:1740-1745.

Lee NM, Brady CW. Liver disease in pregnancy. *World J Gastroenterol*. 2009;15:897-906.

Leese T, Farges O, Bismuth H. Liver cell adenomas. A 12-year surgical experience from a specialist hepato-biliary unit. *Ann Surg*. 1988;208:558-564.

Levy C, Zein CO, Gomez J, et al. Prevalence and predictors of esophageal varices in patients with primary biliary cirrhosis. *Clin Gastroenterol Hepatol*. 2007;5:803-808.

Li CP, Lee FY, Hwang SJ, et al.. Treatment of mastalgia with tamoxifen in male patients with liver cirrhosis: a randomized crossover study. *Am J Gastroenterol*. 2000;95:1051-1055.

Lindor KD, Gershwin ME, Poupon R, Kaplan M, Bergasa NV, Heathcote EJ. Primary biliary cirrhosis. *Hepatology*. 2009;50:291-308.

Liu LU, Schiano TD. Long-term care of the liver transplant recipient. *Clin Liver Dis*. 2007;11:397-416.

Liu S, Chan KW, Wang B, Qiao L. Fibrolamellar hepatocellular carcinoma. *Am J Gastroenterol*. 2009;104:2617-2624; quiz 2625.

Llovet JM, Fuster J, Bruix J. Intention-to-treat analysis of surgical treatment for early hepatocellular carcinoma: resection versus transplantation. *Hepatology*. 1999;30:1434-1440.

Llovet JM, Ricci S, Mazzaferro V, et al. Sorafenib in advanced hepatocellular carcinoma. *N Engl J Med*. 2008;359:378-390.

Lok AS, McMahon BJ. Chronic hepatitis B: update 2009. *Hepatology*. 2009;50:661-662.

Longeville JH, de la Hall P, Dolan P, et al. Treatment of a giant haemangioma of the liver with Kasabach-Merritt syndrome by orthotopic liver transplant: a case report. *HPB Surg*. 1997;10:159-162.

Lum G. Significance of low serum alkaline phosphatase activity in a predominantly adult male population. *Clin Chem*. 1995;41:515-518.

Malinchoc M, Kamath PS, Gordon FD, Peine CJ, Rank J, ter Borg PC. A model to predict poor survival in patients undergoing transjugular intrahepatic portosystemic shunts. *Hepatology*. 2000;31:864-871.

Marcellin P, Forns X, Goeser T, et al. Telaprevir is effective given every 8 or 12 hourse with ribavirin and peginterferon alfa-2a or -2b to patients with chronic hepatitis C. *Gastroenterol*. 2011;140:459-468.

Marchesa P, Lashner BA, Lavery IC, et al. The risk of cancer and dysplasia among ulcerative colitis patients with primary sclerosing cholangitis. *Am J Gastroenterol*. 1997;92:1285-1288.

Mas-Coma S. Epidemiology of fascioliasis in human endemic areas. *J Helminthol*. 2005;79:207-216.

Mazzaferro V, Regalia E, Doci R, et al. Liver transplantation for the treatment of small hepatocellular carcinomas in patients with cirrhosis. *N Engl J Med*. 1996;334:693-699.

McDowell Torres D, Stevens R, Gurakar A. Acute liver failure: a management challenge for the practicing gastroenterologist. *Gastroenterol Hepatol*. 2010;6:444-450.

McLaran CJ, Bett JH, Nye JA, Halliday JW. Congestive cardiomyopathy and haemochromatosis—rapid progression possibly accelerated by excessive ingestion of ascorbic acid. *Aust N Z J Med*. 1982;12:187-188.

McTigue KM, Harris R, Hemphill B, et al. Screening and interventions for obesity in adults: summary of the evidence for the U.S. Preventive Services Task Force. *Ann Intern Med*. 2003;139:933-949.

Meguro M, Soejima Y, Taketomi A, et al. Living donor liver transplantation in a patient with giant hepatic hemangioma complicated by Kasabach-Merritt syndrome: report of a case. *Surg Today*. 2008;38:463-468.

Mendes FD, Kim WR, Pedersen R, Therneau T, Lindor KD. Mortality attributable to cholestatic liver disease in the United States. *Hepatology*. 2008;47:1241-1247.

Menon KV, Angulo P, Weston S, Dickson ER, Lindor KD. Bone disease in primary biliary cirrhosis: independent indicators and rate of progression. *J Hepatol*. 2001;35:316-323.

Moore KP, Wong F, Gines P, et al. The management of ascites in cirrhosis: report on the consensus conference of the International Ascites Club. *Hepatology*. 2003;38:258-266.

Moreno-Otero R, Trapero-Marugan M. Extrahepatic conditions associated with primary biliary cirrhosis. *Hepatology*. 2010;51:713.

Morgan M, Keeffe EB. Diagnosis and treatment of chronic hepatitis B: 2009 update. *Minerva Gastroenterol Dietol*. 2009;55:5-22.

Morrison ED, Brandhagen DJ, Phatak PD, et al. Serum ferritin level predicts advanced hepatic fibrosis among U.S. patients with phenotypic hemochromatosis. *Ann Intern Med*. 2003;138:627-633.

Morris-Stiff G, Coles G, Moore R, Jurewicz A, Lord R. Abdominal wall hernia in autosomal dominant polycystic kidney disease. *Br J Surg*. 1997;84:615-617.

O'Grady JG, Alexander GJ, Hayllar KM, Williams R. Early indicators of prognosis in fulminant hepatic failure. *Gastroenterology*. 1989;97:439-445.

O'Shea RS, Dasarathy S, McCullough AJ. Alcoholic liver disease. *Am J Gastroenterol*. 2010;105:14-32; quiz 33.

Ostapowicz G, Fontana RJ, Schiodt FV, et al. Results of a prospective study of acute liver failure at 17 tertiary care centers in the United States. *Ann Intern Med*. 2002;137:947-954.

Pachera S, Nishio H, Yamada H, et al. Superextended hepatectomy for resection of multiple giant hemangiomas: report of a case. *Surg Today*. 2009;39:452-455.

Palma DT, Fallon MB. The hepatopulmonary syndrome. *J Hepatol*. 2006;45:617-625.

Papatheodoridis GV, Manolakopoulos S. EASL clinical practice guidelines on the management of chronic hepatitis B: the need for liver biopsy. *J Hepatol*. 2009;51:226-227.

Pardi DS, Loftus EV Jr, Kremers WK, Keach J, Lindor KD. Ursodeoxycholic acid as a chemopreventive agent in patients with ulcerative colitis and primary sclerosing cholangitis. *Gastroenterology*. 2003;124:889-893.

Passarella M, Fallon MB, Kawut SM. Portopulmonary hypertension. *Clin Liver Dis*. 2006;10:653-663, x.

Pastor CM, Schiffer E. Therapy insight: hepatopulmonary syndrome and orthotopic liver transplantation. *Nat Clin Pract Gastroenterol Hepatol*. 2007;4:614-621.

Pawlotsky JM. EASL Clinical Practice Guidelines. *J Hepatol*. 2009;50:243.

Pietrangelo A. Hereditary hemochromatosis: pathogenesis, diagnosis, and treatment. *Gastroenterology*. 2010;139:393-408, 408 e1-2.

Polson J, Lee WM. AASLD position paper: the management of acute liver failure. *Hepatology*. 2005;41:1179-1197.

Poordad F, McCone J Jr, Bacon BR, et al. Boceprevir for untreated chronic HCV genotype 1 infection. *N Engl J Med*. 2011;364:1195-1206.

Riely CA. Liver disease in the pregnant patient. *Am J Gastroenterol*. 1999;94:1728-1732.

Roberts EA, Schilsky ML. Diagnosis and treatment of Wilson disease: an update. *Hepatology*. 2008;47:2089-2111.

Roberts JP, Venook A, Kerlan R, Yao F. Hepatocellular carcinoma: ablate and wait versus rapid transplantation. *Liver Transpl*. 2010;16:925-929.

Rubin RA, Mitchell DG. Evaluation of the solid hepatic mass. *Med Clin North Am*. 1996;80:907-928.

Runyon BA. Care of patients with ascites. *N Engl J Med*. 1994;330:337-342.

Sanchez-Tapias JM, Costa J, Mas A, Bruguera M, Rodes J. Influence of hepatitis B virus genotype on the long-term outcome of chronic hepatitis B in western patients. *Gastroenterology*. 2002;123:1848-1856.

Sandhu BS, Sanyal AJ. Pregnancy and liver disease. *Gastroenterol Clin North Am*. 2003;32:407-436, ix.

Sansonno D, Gesualdo L, Manno C, Schena FP, Dammacco F. Hepatitis C virus-related proteins in kidney tissue from hepatitis C virus-infected patients with cryoglobulinemic membranoproliferative glomerulonephritis. *Hepatology*. 1997;25:1237-1244.

Sanyal AJ. AGA technical review on nonalcoholic fatty liver disease. *Gastroenterology*. 2002;123:1705-1725.

Scheff RT, Zuckerman G, Harter H, Delmez J, Koehler R. Diverticular disease in patients with chronic renal failure due to polycystic kidney disease. *Ann Intern Med*. 1980;92:202-204.

Schiodt FV, Rochling FA, Casey DL, Lee WM. Acetaminophen toxicity in an urban county hospital. *N Engl J Med*. 1997;337:1112-1117.

Schmidt LE, Dalhoff K. Alpha-fetoprotein is a predictor of outcome in acetaminophen-induced liver injury. *Hepatology*. 2005;41:26-31.

Sharma MP, Dasarathy S, Verma N, Saksena S, Shukla DK. Prognostic markers in amebic liver abscess: a prospective study. *Am J Gastroenterol*. 1996;91:2584-2588.

Shetty K, Rybicki L, Brzezinski A, Carey WD, Lashner BA. The risk for cancer or dysplasia in ulcerative colitis patients with primary sclerosing cholangitis. *Am J Gastroenterol*. 1999;94:1643-1649.

Soetikno RM, Lin OS, Heidenreich PA, Young HS, Blackstone MO. Increased risk of colorectal neoplasia in patients with primary sclerosing cholangitis and ulcerative colitis: a meta-analysis. *Gastrointest Endosc*. 2002;56:48-54.

Sorokin A, Brown JL, Thompson PD. Primary biliary cirrhosis, hyperlipidemia, and atherosclerotic risk: a systematic review. *Atherosclerosis*. 2007;194:293-299.

Spiegel BM, DeRosa VP, Gralnek IM, Wang V, Dulai GS. Testing for celiac sprue in irritable bowel syndrome with predominant diarrhea: a cost-effectiveness analysis. *Gastroenterology*. 2004;126:1721-1732.

Spiegel BM, Targownik L, Dulai GS, Karsan HA, Gralnek IM. Endoscopic screening for esophageal varices in cirrhosis: Is it ever cost effective? *Hepatology*. 2003;37:366-377.

Springer JE, Cole DE, Rubin LA, et al. Vitamin D-receptor genotypes as independent genetic predictors of decreased bone mineral density in primary biliary cirrhosis. *Gastroenterology*. 2000;118:145-151.

Stratopoulos C, Papakonstantinou A, Terzis I, et al. Changes in liver histology accompanying massive weight loss after gastroplasty for morbid obesity. *Obes Surg*. 2005;15:1154-1160.

Sturniolo GC, Molokhia MM, Shields R, Turnberg LA. Zinc absorption in Crohn's disease. *Gut*. 1980;21:387-391.

Swanson KL, Wiesner RH, Krowka MJ. Natural history of hepatopulmonary syndrome: impact of liver transplantation. *Hepatology*. 2005;41:1122-1129.

Swanson KL, Wiesner RH, Nyberg SL, Rosen CB, Krowka MJ. Survival in portopulmonary hypertension: Mayo Clinic experience categorized by treatment subgroups. *Am J Transplant*. 2008;8:2445-2453.

Sylvestre PB, Batts KP, Burgart LJ, Poterucha JJ, Wiesner RH. Recurrence of primary biliary cirrhosis after liver transplantation: histologic estimate of incidence and natural history. *Liver Transpl*. 2003;9:1086-1093.

Targownik LE, Spiegel BM, Dulai GS, Karsan HA, Gralnek IM. The cost-effectiveness of hepatic venous pressure gradient monitoring in the prevention of recurrent variceal hemorrhage. *Am J Gastroenterol*. 2004;99:1306-1315.

Tavill AS. Diagnosis and management of hemochromatosis. *Hepatology*. 2001;33:1321-1328.

Tenner S, Dubner H, Steinberg W. Predicting gallstone pancreatitis with laboratory parameters: a meta-analysis. *Am J Gastroenterol*. 1994;89:1863-1866.

ter Borg MJ, Leemans WF, de Man RA, Janssen HL. Exacerbation of chronic hepatitis B infection after delivery. *J Viral Hepat*. 2008;15:37-41.

Terriff BA, Gibney RG, Scudamore CH. Fatality from fine-needle aspiration biopsy of a hepatic hemangioma. *Am J Roentgenol*. 1990;154:203-204.

Thompson AJ, Muir AJ, Sulkowski MS, et al. Interleukin-28B polymorphism improves viral kinetics and is the strongest pretreatment predictor of sustained virologic response in genotype 1 hepatitis C virus. *Gastroenterology*. 2010;139:120-129 e18.

Thorsen S, Ronne-Rasmussen J, Petersen E, Isager H, Seefeldt T, Mathiesen L. Extra-intestinal amebiasis: clinical presentation in a non-endemic setting. *Scand J Infect Dis*. 1993;25:747-750.

Tillmann HL, Hadem J, Leifeld L, et al. Safety and efficacy of lamivudine in patients with severe acute or fulminant hepatitis B, a multicenter experience. *J Viral Hepat*. 2006;13:256-263.

Toso C, Mentha G, Kneteman NM, Majno P. The place of downstaging for hepatocellular carcinoma. *J Hepatol*. 2010;52:930-936.

Vasan RS, Pencina MJ, Cobain M, Freiberg MS, D'Agostino RB. Estimated risks for developing obesity in the Framingham Heart Study. *Ann Intern Med*. 2005;143:473-480.

Veluru C, Atluri D, Chadalavada R, Burns E, Mullen KD. Skin rash during chronic hepatitis C therapy. *Gastroenterol Hepatol*. 2010;6:323-325.

Vera A, Gunson BK, Ussatoff V, Nightingale P, et al. Colorectal cancer in patients with inflammatory bowel disease after liver transplantation for primary sclerosing cholangitis. *Transplantation*. 2003;75:1983-1988.

Watt KD, Pedersen RA, Kremers WK, Heimbach JK, Charlton MR. Evolution of causes and risk factors for mortality post-liver transplant: results of the NIDDK long-term follow-up study. *Am J Transplant*. 2010;10:1420-1427.

Weibrecht K, Dayno M, Darling C, Bird SB. Liver aminotransferases are elevated with rhabdomyolysis in the absence of significant liver injury. *J Med Toxicol*. 2010;6:294-300.

Wolf G. A history of vitamin A and retinoids. *FASEB J*. 1996;10:1102-1107.

Yang HI, Lu SN, Liaw YF, et al. Hepatitis B e antigen and the risk of hepatocellular carcinoma. *N Engl J Med*. 2002;347:168-174.

Yen TC, Hwang SJ, Wang CC, Lee SD, Yeh SH. Hypercalcemia and parathyroid hormone-related protein in hepatocellular carcinoma. *Liver*. 1993;13:311-315.

Yeoman AD, Al-Chalabi T, Karani JB, et al. Evaluation of risk factors in the development of hepatocellular carcinoma in autoimmune hepatitis: implications for follow-up and screening. *Hepatology*. 2008;48:863-870.

Yu L, Ioannou GN. Survival of liver transplant recipients with hemochromatosis in the United States. *Gastroenterology*. 2007;133:489-495.

Zein CO, Jorgensen RA, Clarke B, et al. Alendronate improves bone mineral density in primary biliary cirrhosis: a randomized placebo-controlled trial. *Hepatology*. 2005;42:762-771.

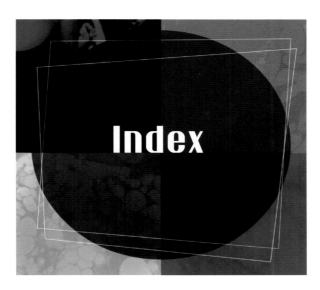

Index

diastase-resistant globules, in alpha-1 antitrypsin deficiency, 189, 194
diclofenac, toxicity of, 54, 58–59
diet
copper avoidance in, 49, 173
vitamin D sources in, 137
dirt, eating, fascioliasis due to, 123–126
disseminated intravascular coagulopathy, in Kasabach-
Merritt syndrome, 13–15
diuretics, for ascites, 109–110
refractory, 174, 176–177
renal toxicity and, 174, 176
diverticulitis, after liver transplantation, 149–150
drainage
of amebic abscess, 106
of hydatid cyst, 213
drug side effects
gynecomastia, 108–110
liver injury
acetaminophen, 81–84, 117–119
amiodarone, 54, 57
anabolic steroids, 55, 60–61
antibiotics, 54, 58–59
azathioprine, 54, 59–60
diclofenac, 54, 58–59
as favorite board topic, 2
hepatocanalicular, 56–58
kava kava, 54, 56
MDMA, 20–21
6-mercaptopurine, 54, 59–60
oral contraceptives, 160
peliosis hepatis, 55, 60–61
statins, 55, 61–63
vitamin A, 55, 61
penicillamine, 171–173
renal toxicity, 3, 174, 176, 178
skin reactions, 68–71
"ductopenia," in primary sclerosing cholangitis, 189, 191
dyspepsia, in hepatic adenoma, 159–160
dyspnea
in hepatopulmonary syndrome, 29–31
in portopulmonary hypertension, 200–201

early response, to hepatitis C therapy, 156–158
early satiety, in polycystic kidney disease, 144–147
echinococcosis, 125–126, 211–213
ecstasy (MDMA) toxicity, 20–21
edema
in HELLP syndrome, 202, 204–206
in hepatopulmonary syndrome, 29–31
in hydatid cyst, 212
in mixed cryoglobulinemia, 174, 178
in portopulmonary hypertension, 200–201
"eggshell" appearance, of hydatid cyst, 212
encephalopathy, hepatic. See hepatic encephalopathy
entecavir, for hepatitis B virus vertical transmission prevention, 39, 40
Entamoeba histolytica, in amebic abscess, 105–108
ERCP (endoscopic retrograde cholangiopancreatography)
for gallstone pancreatitis, 209–210
for recurrent pyogenic cholangitis, 181–182
erythema, palmar, in normal pregnancy, 167–168
erythromycin
for peliosis hepatis, 61
toxicity of, 57–58

esophageal varices
in cirrhosis, 50–53
in normal pregnancy, 166–168
in polycystic kidney disease, 144–147
esophageal vein, in portal circulation, 17–18
ethnic variations. See genetic factors
exertional heat stroke, acute liver failure during, 114–116

fascioliasis, 123–126
fatigue
in acute alcoholic hepatitis, 76–80
in amebic abscess, 105–108
in HELLP syndrome, 202, 204–206
in hepatitis E virus infections, 141–143
in hepatocellular carcinoma, 185–188
in hypothyroidism, 151, 152
in normal pregnancy, 166–168
in overlap syndrome of autoimmune hepatitis and
primary biliary cirrhosis, 139–140
in polymyositis, 91–92
in portopulmonary hypertension, 200–201
fatty liver
in alcohol use, 76-80
in pregnancy, 202–205
in Wilson disease, 47–49
fatty liver disease, nonalcoholic, 99, 103–104, 161–165
ferritin, elevated, in hemochromatosis, 67–68
fever
in hepatitis E virus infections, 141–143
in herpes simplex virus hepatitis, 183–184
in pelvic inflammatory disease, 22–24
penicillamine-induced, 171–173
in typhoid fever, 111–113
fibrolamellar hepatocellular carcinoma, 72–75
fibrosis
in nonalcoholic steatohepatitis, 189, 190
in primary sclerosing cholangitis, 189, 191
fistulas, arteriovenous, 127, 129
Fitz-Hugh-Curtis syndrome, 22–24
"flask-shaped" ulcerations, in amebic abscess, 106–107
flat parasites, 123–126
"florid duct lesion," in primary biliary cirrhosis, 101, 189,
190
flukes, liver, 123–126
flushing, in mastocytosis, 169–170
fluvastatin, 62
focal nodular hyperplasia, vs. hepatocellular carcinoma,
73–75
fundic varices, 16–19
furosemide, for ascites, 108–110, 174, 176–177

gait disturbance, in vitamin E deficiency, 135, 136
gallbladder polyps, in primary sclerosing cholangitis, 121
gallstone pancreatitis, 93–95, 209–210
gastric bypass, for morbid obesity, 164
gastric varices, 16–19
gastroparesis, erythromycin-induced, 57–58
genetic factors
in body mass index, 163
in fatty liver of pregnancy, 202–204
in hepatitis B virus, 40
in hepatitis C virus, 156–158, 197–199
in intrahepatic cholestasis of pregnancy, 202, 203
germander, toxicity of, 56
giant hemangiomas, in Kasabach-Merritt syndrome, 13–15